BEHAVIORAL INTERVENTION IN HEALTH CARE

BEHAVIORAL SCIENCES FOR HEALTH CARE PROFESSIONALS
Michael A. Counte, Series Editor

During the 1970s there was rapid growth in the amount of behavioral science instruction included in the training of physicians, nurses, dentists, pharmacists, and other health care professionals. New faculty members were put on staffs at medical centers, curricula were devised, and on occasion, new departments were created to support a diverse group of behavioral scientists.

The new emphasis on behavioral science in the education of health care professionals and the inclusion of a behavioral science section in certification examinations have generated a need for clinically relevant text materials. This series responds to that need by providing general, yet concise, introductions to common topical areas in behavioral science curricula, linking concepts and theories to clinical practice.

The authors of the series volumes are behavioral scientists with considerable experience in the education of health care professionals. Most of them are also clinicians, and their varied experience enables them to present their topics in a readable fashion. The content of the texts presumes only a very basic knowledge of the behavioral sciences, and emphasis is placed on the practical implications of research findings for health care delivery.

It is our hope that this multivolume approach will allow each instructor to select the books most pertinent to his or her particular curriculum. The division of topics was planned to enhance the overall flexibility of the information being presented.

Forthcoming in This Series

Also of Interest

† Available in hardcover and paperback.

BEHAVIORAL INTERVENTION IN HEALTH CARE

Laura B. Gordon, Ph.D.

Rush Medical College,
Rush–Presbyterian–St. Luke's Medical Center

It has been demonstrated that many medical problems, including insomnia, alcoholism, hypertension, headache, pain, obesity, and asthma, respond readily and reliably to behavior modification techniques. Yet, behavioral intervention has traditionally been a difficult area to assimilate into the medical and nursing curricula. In this text, Dr. Laura B. Gordon presents a behavioral-psychological perspective on intervention in health care, beginning with a definition of behavioral medicine and introducing the related issues of stress and patient compliance.

With an emphasis on how behavioral intervention relates to clinical practice, Dr. Gordon examines such topics as the role of the patient's behavior in the symptom or disease, how the health care professional can identify those who will respond well to individual or family counseling, and the treatment of disease versus the maintenance of health. She concludes with an explanation of the need for less conventional facilities for treating psychophysiological and stress/tension disorders, pointing to the program currently in use at the Dartmouth-Hitchcock Medical Center as one possible alternative approach.

Dr. Laura B. Gordon is assistant professor of psychology and social science at Rush University's College of Medicine and assistant scientist at Rush–Presbyterian–St. Luke's Medical Center in Chicago.

BEHAVIORAL SCIENCES FOR HEALTH CARE PROFESSIONALS

BEHAVIORAL INTERVENTION IN HEALTH CARE

Laura B. Gordon, Ph.D.

Rush Medical College,
Rush–Presbyterian–St. Luke's Medical Center

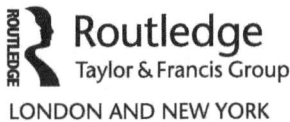
Routledge
Taylor & Francis Group

LONDON AND NEW YORK

Behavioral Sciences for Health Care Professionals

First publishing 1982 by Westview Press, Inc.

Published 2018 by Routledge
52 Vanderbilt Avenue, New York, NY 10017
2 Park Square, Milton Park, Abingdon, Oxon OX14 4RN

Routledge is an imprint of the Taylor & Francis Group, an informa business

Library of Congress Cataloging in Publication Data
Gordon, Laura B.
  Behavioral intervention in health care.
  (Behavioral sciences for health care professionals)
  Includes bibliographies and index.
  1. Medicine and psychology. 2. Health behavior. 3. Behavior modification.
I. Title. II. Series.
R726.5.G67   615.8'51   81-14726
ISBN 0-86531-018-1   AACR2
ISBN 0-86531-019-X (pbk.)

ISBN 13: 978-0-367-01831-3 (hbk)
ISBN 13: 978-0-367-16818-6 (pbk)

To Jerry and Jonathan Marc

CONTENTS

BEHAVIORAL INTERVENTION IN HEALTH CARE

1

INTRODUCTION

This book will illustrate the significance of behavioral intervention in a medical setting by describing medical problems that are essentially behavioral disorders or are determined in part by the behavioral responses of the patient. The cases discussed will provide a basis for understanding the overall role of behavioral intervention in specific health problems like insomnia, alcoholism, headache, obesity, pain, and hypertension. Other common problems such as grief reactions, decompensation, or decline in mental functions as a consequence of aging and various kinds of medical illness, and non-compliance with medically prescribed practices will also be considered. Although behavioral intervention is the main focus of this volume, counseling intervention approaches are also discussed. Frequently they provide necessary alternatives with which the health care professional should be familiar. Psychiatry has traditionally provided information about psychopathology to the medical profession, but it is the goal of this book to underscore the relevance of behavioral medicine to the entire health care field. An extensive bibliography appears at the end of each chapter, and the interested reader is encouraged to pursue these leads for further information.

WHAT IS BEHAVIORAL MEDICINE?

There has been increasing interest in what has been termed health care psychology, the application of behavioral principles to problems of physical health and illness. This approach emphasizes the psychobiology of health and directs attention to the interaction of psychosocial and biological processes in both health and disease. The emergence of behavioral medicine (Miller, 1975) has been a direct consequence of this interest. In general, behavioral medicine involves the application of behavioral principles to a broad range of medical problems beyond those psychological disorders with which clinical psychology has traditionally been concerned. More specifically, behavioral medicine is "an approach to illness states which utilizes assessment techniques to evaluate affective, cognitive, psychophysiologic, behavioral, and environmental aspects of illness and encompasses treatment techniques with a predominantly psychobehavioral component" (Morgan, Kramer, and Gaylor, 1977:88). Behavioral medicine is most concerned with the psychological factors or behavioral contingencies that help maintain or serve to exacerbate the illness process.

It is important to differentiate the behavioral area of medicine from that of psychosomatic medicine. There is a tendency to view them as synonymous, but they are distinctly different. Psychosomatic medicine stresses the etiology and pathogenesis of physical disease. Behavioral medicine is primarily concerned with the prevention and treatment of disease through the use of behavioral techniques. A more complete description of behavioral medicine has been given by Schwartz and Weiss (1977:378): "Behavioral medicine focuses on the development of behavioral science, its knowledge, and techniques in the understanding of physical health and illness, and the application of such knowledge and techniques to diagnosis, prevention, treatment, and rehabilitation." This definition stresses the psychobiological foundations of human behavior and points to their relevance to the fields of clinical psychology, nursing, and medicine.

The focal ideas of behavioral medicine revolve around an individual's susceptibility to illness, ability to cope, and response to the recommended treatment program. Perhaps the most basic tenet of behavioral medicine is that each person is responsible for his own behavior and well-being. The commonplace phrase "it's only psychological" indicates widespread contempt for difficulties having psychological roots or consequences and suggests that psychologically caused problems are somehow equivalent to mental illness. The word "psychological" can be easily misconstrued by patients, suggesting to them that they are relieved of responsibility for their own care. The effects of physical states of illness on the subjective feelings of the patient and on his ability to cope are primary considerations in behavioral medicine. There has been an increasing demand for this sort of health care service due to heightened psychological needs, decreased tolerance for discomfort coupled with expectations of immediate relief, and a generally greater acceptance of disclosure of psychological complaints. Consideration of the psychological and social factors that influence health care will enable the professional to better prepare patients for medical treatment and to facilitate compliance with prescribed behavioral and pharmacological routines. When the approach to a problem takes place in the context of the patient's own behavior and experiences, he is more likely to feel responsible and to take an active role in developing satisfactory, effective coping mechanisms.

The unique psychology of each person must be considered in planning medical care. Psychological factors are especially important in treating chronic diseases that are the contemporary precursors of death. (This is in marked contrast to the early 1900s, when infectious disease was the leading cause of death.) Although current medical education is often geared to acute disease, arranging chronic care for a patient requires knowledge of the patient's psychological state. The use of too many medical specialists, for example, may cause confusion and discontinuity for the patient. Technology has produced a wide variety of drugs, but it has become increasingly difficult for physicians and nurses to persuade patients to comply with prescribed treatment regimens. Behavioral techniques provide one way to encourage compliance. For example, hypertension has been cited repeatedly as a major cause of morbidity and mortality, and although regular use of antihypertensive medication can dramatically lower this risk, a large body of research shows that less than one-half of the patients at risk adhere to medical advice and use their medication as prescribed. Attention to a behavioral component in medical treatment does not by itself ensure compliance with the prescribed treatment program. It is important for the health care professional to consult with other professionals and with their patients to evolve a comprehensive program that maximizes the probability of compliance.

INTERVENTION TECHNIQUES

Intervention techniques in behavioral medicine are based on the principles of learning theory. The key to producing an adequate treatment program is understanding the processes by which an individual learns certain behaviors and the kinds of conditioning that person has been subjected to. The actual relationship between autonomic-visceral and somatic-motor mechanisms may be a matter of controversy (Black, 1968; DiCara, 1970), but it is clear that learning and conditioning do have a systematic effect on the body's physiological, anatomical, and biochemical systems. The impact of these two factors on a person's overall functioning must then be taken into account. A detailed discussion of learning theory is beyond the scope of this book, but a good review can be found in Hilgard and Bower (1966).

The primary belief underlying all behavioral interventions is that a connection exists between the autonomic and voluntary nervous systems and that autonomic processes are far more susceptible to voluntary control than was originally thought. All behavior is subject to the limitations and inclinations of the individual. Maladaptive behaviors are seen as being maintained by current, observable events, and behavioral medicine is concerned with the assessment and treatment of medical or medically related problems caused by those ongoing environmental influences. In the past, medical problems were usually treated with traditional medical prescriptions alone, but now reports of behavioral interventions in medical illness in the literature (Katz and Zlutnick, 1975) suggest growing enthusiasm for including the behavioral approach.

Behavioral intervention is useful for treating many physical, psychological, and psychophysiological disorders. The techniques of behavior modification include progressive relaxation, biofeedback, desensitization, flooding, modeling, aversive therapy, thought stopping, and social skills training. (A description of some routine use of these techniques can be found in Chapter 2.) The key to successful behavioral treatment is the detailed assessment of the patient that should precede every treatment attempt. Every responsible treatment plan usually begins with some kind of assessment, but assessment frequently constitutes the major part of behavioral intervention. Behavioral assessment requires an operational definition of the presenting problem, that is, the way that the problem is manifested behaviorally. Insomnia or overeating are examples of operational definitions. The practitioner must also evaluate the skills the individual will need to acquire before the desired goal behavior can be attained and must look at the environmental factors that are preventing the patient from learning those baseline skills. A functional analysis of behavior must also be conducted in order to learn which environmental factors are maintaining a problem. This functional analysis describes events that precede or follow a specific behavior so that a decision about the utility of a specific behavioral approach can be made.

A total behavioral assessment requires consideration of six major areas: (1) the personality of an individual will affect what illness occurs and how that person will cope with it. People react to the stress of illness with a specific constellation of cognitive, emotional, physiological, and behavioral responses based on their underlying psychological style (Lipowski, 1977; Millon, Green, and Meagher, 1979). (2) Premorbid pessimism influences the course of illness and the recuperative period. For example, premorbid depression has been shown to result in a more prolonged, difficult postoperative period (Boyd, Yeager, and McMillan, 1973). (3) Interpersonal support serves to moderate life stressors (Cobb, 1976). (4) Excessive concern about bodily functions constitutes a major stress and can adversely affect a person's ability to cope with illness (Lucente and Fleck, 1972). (5) Psychological problems underlying the illness state as well as the psychosomatic correlates of a disease must be carefully assessed. (6) And finally, the process of sorting out which patients will respond well or poorly to a medical procedure should lead to methods of classification that will decrease the frequency of poor outcome. All of these variables must be considered for every problem presented in order to allow maximum utility of behavioral techniques that will encourage an individual to learn more appropriate, health-productive behaviors.

ILLNESS PREVENTION

A common misconception is that behavioral medicine is focused on treating health problems, much as traditional medicine is geared to the treatment of disorders. In fact, behavioral medicine is equally involved with preventive measures. Although necessarily this discussion is primarily concerned with treatment, a brief look at prevention is warranted as well. Faulty habits and various maladaptive behaviors or lifestyles are often implicated in the development of certain physical disorders. It is possible to gradually change these habits and lifestyles through programs using behavioral principles, thereby significantly reducing the risk of medical disorder. The way an individual copes with stress may strongly influence his general adjustment and propensity to physical illness. For example, the person who overeats as a means of coping with chronic anxiety is likely to become obese, which will not only result in poor self-esteem but may also contribute to a number of undesirable physical complications.

Consider the relationship of Type A and Type B personalities to coronary heart disease (Jenkins, Zyganski, and Rosenman, 1978). The classic Type A individual is described as hostile, competitive, unable to relax, pressured, loud, and impatient. Much research has focused on the use of behavior modification techniques to alter various aspects of Type A behavior (Suinn and Richardson, 1971; Suinn, 1974; Suinn, 1975a). There is as yet little evidence to demonstrate that such interventions can produce long-term change, and there is no current data to indicate that altering Type A behaviors will reduce the incidence or recurrence of coronary heart disease. However, the work of Peterson, Keith, and Wilcox (1962) and Clark et al. (1975) reveals that cholesterol does increase during periods of stress. A program for prevention of heart disease, then, might well focus on the alteration of dietary habits or on reducing stress. In view of society's reinforcements of Type A behavior (such as material success and media glorification of achievers), the modification or reduction of such behavior is exceedingly difficult (Zeldow, 1980). Nevertheless, the techniques of behavioral medicine allow the health care professional to identify the psychosocial variables that predispose a patient to stress and eventual medical difficulty and to integrate them into a corrective health regimen.

The skills needed for coping with stress must, of course, be viewed in an environmental context. During each contact, the practitioner can focus on the specific interpersonal, personal, and social skills needed by a patient at that time. Determining whether the necessary skills are available to the patient or whether the patient's environment can facilitate the learning of these skills helps the practitioner assess the patient's ongoing functioning and begin programs for behavior changes that will be conducive to health. Optimally this evaluation should be made before any actual medical illness is brought on by faulty habits or high-risk lifestyles. Certainly the economic advantages of such a preventive approach are obvious, given the costs—physical, mental, and material—of treating chronic illness.

STRESS REDUCTION

The way people cope with stress definitely affects their lifestyles and, hence, their potential state of health (Bieliauskas, 1981).

Physical stress is easily pinpointed. Although the precise manifestations may vary with the particular way that each person routinely
copes with stress, they most often include heightened muscle tension, increased heart rate, sweating, rapid respiration, and excessive
hormonal release. Seligman (1975) has demonstrated that an individual who feels out of control experiences decreased motivation
to respond and a heightening of underlying emotionality. The result
is what he terms "learned helplessness." Stress is greater under conditions of helplessness, where only the futility of action is perceived.
Engel (1971) expanded upon this notion and cited data from 170
cases of sudden death indicating that negative psychological states
(such as the depression that often results from the loss of a close
friend or relative) preceded the subjects' deaths. Methodological problems in the study do not permit us to conclude that psychological
stress causes death, but stressors do clearly tax existing defensive
styles, thereby increasing the degree of stress. It is conceivable that a
patient with a major disorder who is subjected to psychological stress
he is not equipped to manage may be at greater risk. Practitioners of
behavioral medicine must consider seriously the stressful events and
circumstances that may interfere with a patient's ability to cope and
contribute to further medical difficulties. Adequate preparation for
unpleasant or painful medical procedures will help patients feel in
better control of themselves and will thereby facilitate stress reduction. Advance information will also make it easier for patients to comply with the medical regimen set out for them.

THE ROLE OF BEHAVIORAL INTERVENTION IN
MEDICAL PRACTICE

In the beginning, behavioral techniques belonged to the domain
of clinical psychologists, but they are now suitable for application to
many medical disorders and to behaviors with health consequences
that are not classified as medical disorders by themselves (for example, obesity or pain). Informed health care professionals can
gather extensive information about behavior as it relates to illness,
health, and potential medical interventions. An understanding of the
psychosocial factors that underlie the development or exacerbation
of various physical complaints and awareness of those personality
traits that will maximize the efficacy of treatment are two valuable
tools provided by the behavioral science approach. In addition,
health care professionals who are especially interested in compliance

with a prescribed medical regimen, with the concept of health-related behavior changes that underlie a preventive model of health care, and with the impact of life stressors on physical illness will find behavioral medicine a highly exciting, relevant field.

BIBLIOGRAPHY

Bandura, A. *Principles of behavior modification.* New York: Holt, Rinehart and Winston, 1969.

Behavioral medicine: An emergent field. *Science,* 1980, 29:479–481.

Bieliauskas, L. A. *Stress and its relationship to health and illness.* Boulder, Colorado: Westview Press, 1981.

Black, A. M. Operant conditioning of autonomic responses. *Conditioned Reflex,* 1968, 3:130.

Blackwell, B. Treatment adherence. *British Journal of Psychiatry,* 1976, 129: 513–531.

Boyd, I., Yeager, M., and McMillan, M. Personality styles in the postoperative course. *Psychosomatic Medicine,* 1973, 35:23–40.

Clark, D. A., Arnold, E. L., Foulds, E. L., Brown, D. M., Eastmead, D. R., and Parry, E. M. Serum urate and cholesterol levels in Air Force Academy cadets. *Aviation Space and Environmental Medicine,* 1975, 46:1044–1048.

Cobb, S. Presidential address – 1976: Social support of a moderator of life stress. *Psychosomatic Medicine,* 1976, 38:300–314.

Davidson, P. O., and Davidson, S. M. *Behavioral medicine: Changing health lifestyles.* New York: Brunner/Mazel, 1980.

DiCara, L. V. Learning in the autonomic nervous system. *Scientific American,* 1970, 220:30–39.

Engel, G. Sudden and rapid death during psychological stress, folklore or folk wisdom? *Annals of Internal Medicine,* 1971, 74:771.

_____. *Psychological development in health and disease.* Philadelphia: W. B. Saunders, 1967.

Goldfried, M. P., and Davison, G. C. *Clinical behavior therapy.* New York: Holt, Rinehart and Winston, 1976.

Hilgard, E. R., and Bower, G. H. *Theories of Learning.* New York: Appleton-Century-Crofts, 1966.

Jenkins, C. Social and epidemiological factors in psychosomatic disease. *Psychiatric Annals,* 1972, 1:8–21.

_____. Assessment of the coronary prone behavior pattern. In T. Dembroski (Ed.), *Proceedings of the forum on coronary prone behavior* (Washington, D.C.: Department of Health, Education and Welfare Publication No.

[NIH] 78-1451, 1977), pp. 104–126.

Jenkins, C., Zyganski, S., and Rosenman, D. Coronary prone behavior: One pattern or several. *Psychosomatic Medicine,* 1978, 40:25–43.

Katz, R., and Zlutnick, R. *Behavior therapy and health care: Principles and applications.* New York: Pergamon Press, 1975.

Lipowski, F. J. Psychosomatic medicine in the 70's: An overview. *American Journal of Psychiatry,* 1977, 134:233–234.

Lucente, F. E., and Fleck, S. A study of hospitalization anxiety in 408 medical and surgical patients. *Psychosomatic Medicine,* 1972, 34:304–312.

Miller, N. Behavioral medicine as a new frontier: Opportunities and dangers. In J. M. Weiss (Ed.), *Proceedings of the National Heart and Lung Institute and working conference on health behavior: Bayse, Virginia, May 12–15, 1975* (Department of Health, Education, and Welfare Publication No. [NIH] 76-868) (Washington, D.C.: Government Printing Office, 1975).

Millon, T., Green, C. J., and Meagher, R. The MCMI: A new inventory for the psychodiagnostician in medical settings. *Professional Psychology,* 1979, 529–539.

Morgan, C. D., Kramer, E., and Gaylor, M. The behavioral medicine unit: A new facility. *Comprehensive Psychiatry,* 1977, 20:79–89.

Peterson, J. E., Keith, R. A., and Wilcox, A. A. Hourly changes in serum cholesterol concentration. Effects of the anticipation of stress. *Circulation,* 1962, 25:798–803.

Pomerleau, O. F., and Brady, J. P. (Eds.). *Behavioral medicine: Theory and practice.* Baltimore: Williams and Wilkins, 1979.

Rosenman, R. M., and Friedman, M. Modifying Type A behavior pattern. *Journal of Psychosomatic Research,* 1979, 21:323–333.

Roskies, E., Spevack, M., Surkis, A., Cohen, C., and Gilman, S. Changing the coronary prone (Type A) behavior pattern in a non-clinical population. *Journal of Behavioral Medicine,* 1978, 1:201–217.

Schwartz, G. E., and Weiss, S. M. What is behavior modification? *Psychosomatic Medicine,* 1977, 39:377–381.

Seligman, M. *Helplessness.* San Francisco: W. H. Freeman, 1975.

Suinn, R. M. Behavioral rehearsal training for ski racers. *Behavior Therapy,* 1972, 3:519.

———. Behavioral therapy for cardiac patients. *Behavior Therapy,* 1974, 5: 569–571.

———. Anxiety management training for general anxiety. In R. Suinn and R. Weigel (Eds.), *The innovative therapist: Creative and critical contributions* (New York: Harper & Row, 1975a), pp. 32–60.

———. The cardiac stress management program for Type A patients. *Cardiac Rehabilitation,* 1975b, 5(4):95–99.

Suinn, R. M., and Bloom, L. J. Anxiety management training for pattern A behavior. *Journal of Behavioral Medicine,* 1978, 1:25–37.

Suinn, R., and Richardson, F. Anxiety management training: A non-specific behavior therapy system for anxiety control. *Behavior Therapy,* 1971, 1:498.

Williams, R. G., and Gentry, W. D. *Behavioral approaches to medical treatment.* Cambridge, Massachusetts: Ballinger, 1977.

Winefield, M. R., and Peay, M. Y. *Behavioral science in medicine.* Baltimore: University Park Press, 1980.

Wolpe, J. *The practice of behavior therapy.* New York: Pergamon Press, 1969.

Zeldow, P. Fundamentals of behavior: Syllabus for lecture on personality adjustment. Unpublished manuscript, Rush Medical College, Chicago, 1980.

CHANGING BEHAVIOR

BEHAVIOR MODIFICATION PROCEDURES

Goals of Modification

The primary aim of behavioral intervention is to alter patterns of behavior. Changing maladaptive lifestyles that encourage the development or enhancement of medical illness and using psychological intervention to facilitate standard medical care are two specific goals. Appropriate behaviors are to be instituted and strengthened; maladaptive behaviors are to be minimized or, if possible, eliminated altogether. It is also important to teach effective coping mechanisms to people facing medical illness. Research has shown that a person's style of coping with stress affects overall morale and somatic health more than the frequency of stress episodes (Goldfried and Goldfried, 1975; Murphy and Moriarty, 1976). Weisman and Worden (1975) have stated that cancer patients with an adequate social support system are more likely to be in good spirits and to have a better survival rate than those who are isolated. In addition to the stress inherent in medical illness, stress may be created by a person's perceived inadequacy in managing aspects of the environment to his own satisfaction or to that of significant others (Davidson and Davidson, 1980). Any perceived inadequacy may seem far worse if the illness is debilitating and reduces the patient's ability to cope. In such cases, teaching the patients new definitions of the behaviors underlying their perceptions and encouraging them to set more suitable goals for themselves is indicated.

Perhaps the most common misconception in the field of behavior modification is that only the overt behavior of the individual is important. This mistaken notion has resulted in widespread negative appraisal of the technique. Critics say that behavioral intervention techniques ignore the complexities of human development and behavior. However, even though behavioral change may at first glance appear to be a relatively simple task, it actually requires a multifaceted assessment of the nature of the behavior in question, the motivation of the patient to change, and the implications of that behavioral change for the patient. While behavioral approaches include an "emphasis on observable and objective assessment" (Williams and Gentry, 1977:3), evaluation of the patient-environment interaction is essential. This entails a consideration of factors outside treatment that affect and are influenced by the patient's behavior, as well as a careful analysis of the characteristics of the health care professional as they interact with those of the patient. An example of this interaction is the influence of the "expert" status attributed to the health care worker on a patient's motivation to change and the outcome of the intervention. It is essential that the patient and healer share a similar belief system; that is, they should agree that intervention is needed. Without this agreement it is probable that few, if any, effective alterations in behavior can be made. Whatever change does occur will probably not be generalized from the treatment setting to the natural environment of the patient; the goals of the intervention will be blocked and the value of the "new behavior" will be short-lived.

Self-Management Procedures

Behavioral intervention is based on the premise that the management and prevention of some medical and medically related disorders can be consciously controlled by the individual. The notion of self-control began to interest behavioral science researchers in the early 1970s. A brief account of self-management as a behavioral intervention follows; for more detail, see Goldfried and Merbaum (1973), Mahoney and Arnkoff (1978), Mahoney and Thoreson (1974), and Thoreson and Mahoney (1974) for more extensive reviews.

Self-monitoring entails the observation by the individual of explicit behaviors. The patient is initially asked to keep a diary of behaviors relating to the focal problem defined in operational terms by the patient and health care professional. For example, if the maladaptive behavior is overeating, the patient might be asked to keep a log of all foods eaten during a period of time, including the hours at which the eating occurred. Following practice with this preliminary task, more demanding self-monitoring skills, such as recording thoughts, feelings, and events preceding the urge to eat, would be added. It is necessary to teach the patient how to monitor his behavior, as the choice of target behaviors depends on what particular information is desired. Which behaviors actually are logged may change as hypotheses about the problem behavior are generated and altered. Several recording techniques, including automatic counting devices and paper-and-pencil methods, are available; the patient should select the most convenient tool. In the example cited above, qualitative information about the type of food eaten, about cues antecedent to the eating behavior, and about subsequent thoughts is obtained from the self-monitoring data. The accuracy of self-reporting can be maximized by clearly specifying the target behavior, emphasizing the need for accuracy, and choosing a suitable self-monitoring device. Self-monitoring should be practiced prior to starting a program and should be regularly supervised by the health care professional. The effort required to ensure that self-monitoring is done regularly and properly is worthwhile: The act of recording one's behavior alone can result in significant behavior change.

The effective use of self-monitoring as a tool for behavior modification requires motivation and honesty on the part of the patient. The approach is particularly helpful for patients, such as hypertensives, who are often noncompliant with a medical treatment program because they may feel no acute discomfort if they do not comply. Although self-monitoring is a promising technique, there are no formal reports of long-term or consistent effectiveness.

Goal Specification

This technique is designed to facilitate self-regulation (Kalb, Winter, and Berlew, 1968). It requires precise specification of goals and the means used to attain these goals. The health care worker should take particular care to help the patient set reasonable goals and prevent further psychological distress (Beck, 1976; Meichenbaum, 1977). Both excessively high goals and self-defeating notions – patients' beliefs that behavioral intervention will not work – are to be avoided with the goal specification technique. This approach has a cognitive-behavioral orientation that allows it to be easily used with other approaches.

Cueing Strategies

Social, physical, and psychological events – antecedents – precipitate behavior. The view that a response depends on the configuration of stimuli preceding it has led to attempts at self-control to restrict, modify, or eliminate maladaptive behavior. Cueing strategies focus on the relationship between stimulus and response. Research has shown that a response to a stimulus is dependent upon one's perception of it: Wooley (1972) demonstrated that the different responses of obese and thin people to the same food are a function of whether the food is perceived as having a high or low calorie count. Obese people perceive a food as low in calories; thin people see the same food as high in calories. Intervention based on this approach requires changing the antecedents of behavior so as to increase the probability of a more adaptive response. A common example is the stimulus control program used to treat insomnia (Bootzin, 1972). It requires patients to alter behaviors that cue sleep. They must keep regular bedtime and morning waking hours, avoid daytime napping, and use bed only for nighttime sleep. These procedures in turn effect a positive change in the maladaptive response of insomnia.

Modification of Incentives

Rewards are effective in the development and maintenance of desired behavior (Mahoney and Arnkoff, 1978; Thoreson and Mahoney, 1974). One can certainly be rewarded as a result of imposing strict standards of behavior on oneself; for example, the characteristic driving nature of the Type A personality results in material gain, which reinforces the original activity. It is more helpful, however, to teach patients more appropriate self-reinforcement behavior that is rewarded by both tangible and private rewards (e.g., thoughts). In addition, establishment of social supports helps people to achieve meaningful self-reward. Research on obesity suggests that social support is crucial in gaining the self-control necessary to lose weight (Brownell et al., 1978). Including self-rewards for achieving an appropriate or desired goal is also a useful technique in increasing compliance with a prescribed medical program.

Rehearsal

Systematic practice of a response helps to reduce the anxiety that may be initially associated with the response. In rehearsal, the tasks to be practiced are arranged in order of increasing difficulty by the health care professional and patient. Rehearsal can be overt or covert. Overt rehearsal is enacted in vivo (in reality), and the consequences of a particular behavior are quickly apparent. Covert rehearsal requires one to practice a response using imagery (Kazdin and Wilson, 1976). The refinement of performance, the experience of efficacy and self-mastery, preparation for potential problems that are currently unknown, and the development of important coping skills are valuable aspects of the rehearsal approach.

Relaxation and Biofeedback Training

Relaxation plays a major role in facilitating biofeedback training; at the same time it is biofeedback's primary goal. Miller (1969) demonstrated in his classical work that involuntary responses of the autonomic nervous system that were once thought to be outside consciousness could actually be conditioned and put under an individual's active control. Relaxation is an aspect of most behavioral forms of interventions. It is the most important treatment factor in a variety of psychophysiological and stress-related disorders. Most people are already aware of the need for "relaxation," but providing the subject with feedback about the quality of the process actually facilitates relaxation (Budzynski and Stoyva, 1969; Green, Green, and Walters, 1970). Progressive muscular relaxation involves learning to relax, in a conscious stepwise fashion, various muscles and muscle groups by imagining pleasant, calming visual scenes while engaging in controlled deep breathing. It provides autonomic control skills that help one to cope with the muscle tension that is symptomatic of anxiety. The growing market for audiotapes of self-help relaxation procedures for a variety of difficulties, including insomnia and anxiety, shows that this approach is popular.

Recently there have been significant advances in understanding the role of the environment and behavior in the regulation of physiological processes. Endless numbers of papers and books have been published on this subject (Barber et al., 1971a, 1971b). Miller (1969) initially proved that visceral response could be shaped; later studies of biofeedback widened the scope of behavioral models in research on physiological functions and emotional states. There was renewed interest in the behavioral etiology of psychophysiological disorders.

Biofeedback entails the application of operant conditioning techniques—the use of positive and negative reinforcements that depend upon selected physiological processes and the learning process that ensues from the control of visceral somatomotor and central nervous system activities. Feedback of biological information about various psychophysiological functions is externally provided by a technical device, which describes specific internal functions. A systematic investigation of the effects of environmental stimuli that depend upon behavior change is conducted. The physiological response of interest must be recorded, measured, or counted. When the focal response occurs in biofeedback (e.g., decreased muscle activity), a reinforcer is delivered in the form of a stimulus, most often a tape, which varies with the quality of the response. The subject thus obtains information about the quality of a response immediately following the response. Biofeedback teaches one to control physiological responses that were previously considered involuntary and automatic. It helps the patient to develop better coping skills. Relaxation has been combined effectively with biofeedback in the treatment of anxiety disorders (Sargent, Green, and Walters, 1972, 1973; Wickramasekera, 1973), hypertension (Patel and North, 1975), and phobias (Wickramasekera, 1973). Budzynski and Stoyva (1969, 1973) gave information to subjects about the level of muscle tension as detected by psychophysiological evaluation. Relaxing these patients and using biofeedback to demonstrate the quality of the relaxation process led to a faster rate of improvement of the original symptom.

Three general issues are paramount in the use of biofeedback and relaxation: (1) achieving the optimal conditions for teaching self-control and mastery of autonomic functions; (2) maximizing the potential for behavior change; and (3) retaining good control and generalization of this response when external feedback signals are no longer received. Disorders entailing precise complaints that are expressed in specific parts of the body and that are not under the control of the patient (e.g., headaches, low back pain) lend themselves to biofeedback treatment. Preliminary evaluations of the flexibility and variability of the functions in question and the appropriateness of biofeedback for each prospective patient must be conducted. The time and effort required by patient and therapist should be commensurate with the expected result: A gradual, stepwise process emphasizing self-control may be appropriate for some people, while those who are more passive and oriented toward immediate gratification might be more efficiently managed with medication.

Patient motivation has a highly significant effect on the outcome of biofeedback and relaxation. Yet, it is not routinely considered in most initial assessments, probably because of the stereotypical view that these intervention techniques are strictly behavioral in focus and ignore cognition altogether. However, it is clear that if the patient does not experience the symptom as aversive or dangerous, he may not be motivated to alter it. For example, although hypertension may be accompanied by changes in physical status and lead to substantial medical deterioration, often it is not manifested in a concrete way to the patient and is prematurely dismissed as inconsequential. Thus, compliance with treatment programs for hypertension is notoriously low. Secondary gain, or the use of symptoms to achieve gratification of needs by other people, may affect motivation to eliminate a symptom. A person may feel that others are more responsive to him when he is sick; when he must take a more dominant stance, he may experience anxiety. It is noteworthy that the bulk of clinical and experimental work with biofeedback and relaxation has been done with highly motivated, educated people. The precise relationship of such patient variables as socioeconomic status, age, intelligence, overall psychosocial adjustment, and the setting of the biofeedback treatment to the outcome of the treatment has not yet been determined.

The nature of the feedback signals can also affect one's response. For example, auditory signals seem to be more effective than visual signals in reducing forehead muscle tension (Schneiderman, Weiss, and Engel, 1979). With practice, a subject can learn to change autonomic response (muscle spasm); he has then achieved control over functions that were previously under the control of the autonomic nervous system.

Can a patient successfully apply responses learned in biofeedback training to relaxed, everyday situations? This issue is much debated among health professionals. Some people in fact apply their biofeedback-trained responses to daily activities, but individual differences in personality, motivation, and the severity of the original problem all influence the degree to which they are successful. Personal lifestyles may conflict with the goal of therapy. For example, hypertension is apt to decrease during the week and increase on weekends if the patient tends to drink more alcohol on weekends. Although drinking is clearly antitherapeutic, it is likely to continue if it is an important aspect of the patient's lifestyle and reinforces aspects of that lifestyle that the patient perceives as gratifying.

Biofeedback is an appropriate intervention for physical disorders that worsen with emotional or environmental stress. Medication may often be valuable in the early stages of biofeedback training to facilitate the initial adjustment and should be considered when necessary. Biofeedback should be utilized only after a patient has received a complete medical evaluation. As most biofeedback training is conducted by psychologists, the health care professional should be prepared to collaborate with the psychologist (or other person conducting biofeedback) on an ongoing basis during the intervention period. Biofeedback training has wide clinical application—for example, in cases of hypertension, cardiac dysfunction, pain, and headache. In addition to the general principles that guide the presentation of biofeedback stimuli, the personality of the individual patient must be considered. The immediate feedback offered in this approach frequently precipitates an increased awareness of maladaptive behaviors; this in turn allows the patient to develop new ways of coping or of altering his lifestyle.

Few follow-up data have been reported on the long-term efficacy of biofeedback and relaxation training. The only consistent finding is that relaxation is the crucial technique. The current lack of standardization of biofeedback stimuli and relaxation procedures makes comparative statements about their relative effectiveness meaningless. Studies comparing relaxation with biofeedback, however, have found that relaxation alone may give as successful a result as biofeedback and relaxation together (Budzynski and Stoyva, 1973; Schneiderman, Weiss, and Engel, 1979). The relationship between a subjective feeling state and the underlying physiological state has not been fully investigated, and most studies have reported a low or negative correlation. Research findings clearly demonstrate that the biofeedback-relaxation training combination is an effective form of intervention in cases of tension headaches, migraine headaches, and hypertension (Beaty and Haynes, 1979; Green, Green, and Walters, 1970; Sargent, Green, and Walters, 1972; Shapiro, Schwartz, and Ferguson, 1977).

In the past there have been reservations about behavioral treatment. The issue of symptom substitution, where new symptoms spontaneously arise from symptoms removed by successful treatment, has not been resolved. In addition, behavioral technology may be misused for purposes that are not in the best interests of the patient (Schwartz, 1973). Schneiderman, Weiss, and Engel (1979:xxiii-xxiv) urged caution in the application of behavioral technology to medical problems.

> When behavioral techniques are used to treat aberrant behavior, contemporary theorists make no assumptions about the underlying diseases which "cause" the atypical behavior. When one is dealing with medical problems where often a great deal is known about the antecedent pathophysiological events, such a formulation is inappropriate. When one attempts to change behavior in a phobic patient, the explicit treatment goal is to change that behavior. However, if one is dealing with a patient who has a history of myocardial disease, the treatment goal is to modify the aberrant response to the extent possible, within the limitations as set by the pathology.

Systematic Desensitization

Wolpe (1958) was the first to develop this approach. In systematic desensitization an individual is gradually exposed to a feared stimulus while he learns to replace the anxiety with a relaxation response. Basing his work on that of Jones (1924), Wolpe found that a fear could be eliminated by learning to associate the feared object or context with a situation capable of producing a pleasant response. The subject is asked first to construct a list of contexts in which the intense fear occurs and then to rank these circumstances from the least to the most feared. The subject also undergoes relaxation training. Systematic desensitization refers to the inhibition of anxiety by a state of relaxation that is incompatible with a fear response. Thus, the context arousing the least anxiety is presented in either a reality (overt) or fantasy (covert) form. When the subject is able to tolerate the presentation of this level of anxiety-provoking images, he continues to the next level, and so on. Practice in vivo is certain to make the process of desensitization more effective. Numerous studies of the application of systematic desensitization support the concept of relaxation as a counter-anxiety state. Lang and Lazovik (1963) showed that relaxation and systematic desensitization together were more effective than relaxation alone in eliminating fear of snakes. Paul (1966) found that systematic desensitization was more successful than psychotherapy in eliminating the fear of public speaking in normal subjects, and Kravetz and Forness (1973) used the procedure to help children learn to visualize freely in the classroom.

Aversive Therapy

This approach creates a connection between an undesirable behavior of the subject and a resulting unpleasant experience. The result is that the behavior drops out of the subject's repertoire. An example of aversive therapy is the taking of Antabuse by alcoholics to prevent them from drinking. Antabuse causes nausea and generalized discomfort (the unpleasant experience) when alcohol is used (undesirable behavior). Aversive therapy is most appropriate for behavior disorders where the behavior is deviant or unconventional but extremely self-rewarding. Aversive therapy frequently requires less time than systematic desensitization, but spontaneous reoccurrence of the undesirable symptom is likely and additional sessions may be periodically necessary to ensure sustained results. Helping the patient to dwell on more acceptable responses while maladaptive responses are being eliminated is a related aspect of the procedure. In the classic work by Voetglin and Lemere et al. (1942), 4000 cases of alcoholism were reviewed. For cases treated with aversive therapy, 50 percent abstained for up to five years and 13 percent for up to twelve years. This rather low improvement rate emphasizes the need for positive reinforcment. It also suggests that when people return to their own environments following treatment, newly learned behaviors are not reinforced and relapse is a potential risk. Interventions like Alcoholics Anonymous (A.A.) attempt to reward new, alternative behaviors while the group reinforces and supports continued involvement in A.A.

Despite much enthusiasm for behavioral intervention, other techniques must at times be utilized as part of a treatment program. Health care personnel have the difficult task of deciding what kind of intervention is best suited to the patient. The following section briefly describes these alternative approaches and the conditions in which they are most appropriate.

COUNSELING APPROACHES

Physical

The illness model considers hospitalization appropriate for people having health care problems with psychological consequences, such as anxiety or depression. Although hospitalization results in the removal of social and community support from the patient, it allows for complete assessment, including the patient's suitability and motivation for a variety of types of intervention, such as chemotherapy and behavioral intervention. In addition, the health care professional has an opportunity to engage the patient in counseling, whether the approach be reeducative, insight-oriented, or cathartic.

Psychodynamic

In this approach it is assumed that psychological problems are caused by intrapsychic conflicts, which are unconscious and result from childhood problems. Gaining insight into these conflicts enables the patient to develop intellectual and emotional awareness of present behavioral or psychological problems. Basic to this approach is the expectation that if a patient gains new understanding of his problems he will change his behavior. The health care professional conducts interviews emphasizing the resolution of conflicts through analysis of past and present interpersonal relationships and through interpretation of dreams. If the patient has medical or medically related disorders, the health care professional must consider the psychodynamic approach as a basis for understanding the patient, at the same time strengthening the patient's unconscious feelings and attitudes, maintaining a reality orientation, and encouraging competence and a sense of mastery over potentially disturbing or stressful events in the patient's life.

Client-Centered

This approach is exemplified by the work of Carl Rogers, who noted that the patient-therapist interaction is the essential aspect of therapy. For treatment to be successful, the therapist must display genuineness, empathy, and unconditional positive regard. The patient will be more apt to realize his potential and develop free of societally imposed constraints if his therapist cares about him. Intervention remains nondirective; the therapist merely facilitates constructive personality change. Goals of the client-centered approach are the expression of feelings, the use of inner experience as a guide to one's own behavior, the interpretation of experience without being rigid or inappropriately concerned with the "right" way, the avoidance of role-playing, the admission that there are problems, and the assumption of responsibility for one's own difficulties. The health care professional merely helps the patient help himself. This approach has given rise to numerous personal growth and encounter groups that provide support for personal growth and understanding. In addition, it has been helpful in training individuals and health care professionals whose jobs demand excellent interpersonal skills. Medical interviewing techniques derive from the client-centered approach.

THE ROLE OF HEALTH CARE PROFESSIONALS

Individuals delivering health care services must be empathic in addition to acting as behavior modifiers. Those who have frequent contact with a patient can best modify patient behavior. Staff nurses are in an excellent position to effect behavioral interventions. For example, they can facilitate elimination of an undesirable response by ignoring a patient when he gives this response, and they can maximize appropriate behaviors by rewarding them. Patients can be expected to meet both subtle and overt demands of the staff. It is not unusual for a patient facing several painful medical procedures to appear passive because he feels he is expected to behave in that manner. Health care professionals must be sensitive to the psychosocial and interpersonal needs of their patients and provide for the consistent management of these needs. Operant conditioning techniques can facilitate recovery of a patient by reinforcing "well behaviors," but the best reinforcement is the approval of the relevant health care people. Lack of attention may result in the extinction of the newly learned appropriate response. The hospital environment breeds a sense of isolation and anxiety on the part of patients. Stimuli like white coats and hospital odors may easily arouse anxiety early in the hospitalization or treatment process. They are likely to maintain a high anxiety level as well; this in turn may interfere with compliance with the prescribed medical regimen and may result in further medical difficulty.

The choice of an appropriate form of intervention, whether

behavioral or counseling, depends on numerous factors, including the nature of the identified problem, the patient's motivation, and his psychological status. A single approach is sometimes most powerful, but a combination of interventions may be most appropriate. For example, obtaining the patient's permission to undergo biofeedback training may require the use of nondirective statements by a genuine, warm health care worker who can allay the patient's anxieties about the procedure and inspire a therapeutic climate of trust and optimism. It is essential that the professional be familiar with a repertoire of techniques and be flexible and comfortable in applying them to a variety of medical or medically related disorders. Certainly, the intervention should be systematically evaluated. The health care professional should assess how far the original goals of intervention have been fulfilled annd how long the improvement has lasted. Although it is often neglected, follow-up is an essential feature of all interventions, one that will ultimately negate or validate them.

BIBLIOGRAPHY

Bandura, A. Influence of models' reinforcement contingencies on the acquisition of imitative responses. *Journal of Personality and Social Psychology,* 1965, 1:589.

Barber, T., DiCara, L., Kamiya, J., Miller, N., Shapiro, D., and Stoyva, J. (Eds.). *Biofeedback and self-control 1970.* Chicago: Aldine, 1971a.

_____. *Biofeedback and self-control reader.* Chicago: Aldine, 1971b.

Beaty, E. T., and Haynes, S. N. Behavioral intervention with muscle contraction headache: A review. *Psychosomatic Medicine,* 1979, 41(2):103–107.

Beck, A. T. *Cognitive therapy and the emotional disorders.* New York: International Universities Press, 1976.

Birk, L. (Ed.). *Biofeedback: Behavioral medicine.* New York: Grune and Stratton, 1973.

Bootzin, R. Stimulus control of isomnia. Presented at a symposium on the treatment of sleep disorders at the annual meeting of the American Psychological Association, Montreal, 1973.

Bootzin, R. R. Stimulus control treatment for insomnia. Paper presented at the 80th annual convention of the American Psychological Association, Honolulu, Hawaii, 1972.

Brockway, B., Kleinmann, G., Edleson, J., et al. Nonaversive procedures and their effect on cigarette smoking. *Addictive Behavior,* 1977, 2:121.

Brownell, K. D., Heckerman, C. L., and Westlake, R. S. Therapist and group contact as variables in the behavioral treatment of obesity. *Journal of Consulting and Clinical Psychology,* 1978, 46(3):593–594.

Budzynski, T. H. Biofeedback procedures in the clinic. In L. Birk (Ed.), *Seminars in psychiatry,* 5 vols. (New York: Grune and Stratton, 1973), 5:461–466.

Budzynski, T. H., and Stoyva, J. M. An instrument for producing deep muscle relaxation by means of analog in information feedback. *Journal of Applied Behavior Analysis,* 1969, 2:231–237.

————. Biofeedback techniques in behavior therapy. In D. Shapiro, T. K. Barber, L. V. DiCara, J. Kamiya, N. E. Miller, and J. Stoyva (Eds.), *Biofeedback and self-control 1972* (Chicago: Aldine, 1973), pp. 293–298.

Burns, R. B. *Psychology for the health professions.* London: International Medical Publishers, 1980.

Cautela, J. R. Treatment of compulsive behavior by covert sensitization. *Psychological Records,* 1968, 16:33–41.

Davidson, P. O., and Davidson, S. M. *Behavioral medicine: Changing health lifestyles.* New York: Brunner/Mazel, 1980.

DiCara, L. V. Learning in the autonomic nervous system. *Scientific American,* 1970, 220:30–39.

D'Zurilla, T. J., and Goldfried, M. R. Problem-solving and behavior modification. *Journal of Abnormal Psychology,* 1971, 78:107–126.

Fordyce, W., Fowler, R., Lehmann, J., and DeLateur, B. Some implications of learning in problems of chronic pain. *Journal of Chronic Disease,* 1968, 21:179.

Goldfried, M. R., and Goldfried, J. P. Cognitive change methods. In F. H. Kanfer and A. P. Goldstein (Eds.), *Helping people change* (New York: Holt, Rinehart and Winston, 1975).

Goldfried, M. R., and Merbaum, M. (Eds.). *Behavior change through self-control.* New York: Holt, Rinehart and Winston, 1973.

Green, E., Green, S., and Walters, D. Voluntary control of internal states: Psychological and psychophysiological. *Journal of Transpersonal Psychology,* 1970, 1:1–26.

Janis, I. *Stress and frustration.* New York: Harcourt Brace Jovanovich, 1971.

Kalb, D. A., Winter, S. K., and Berlew, D. R. Self-directed change: 25 studies. *Journal of Applied Behavioral Science,* 1968: 4:453–476.

Kazdin, A., and Wilson, G. T. *Evaluation of behavior therapy.* Cambridge, Massachusetts: Ballinger, 1976.

Kravetz, R., and Forness, S. The classroom as a desensitizing setting. *Exceptional Child,* 1973, 37:398.

Lang, P. I., and Lazovik, A. D. Experimental desensitization of a phobia. *Journal of Abnormal and Social Psychology.* 1963, 66:519.

Lazarus, A. Multimodal behavioral treatment of depression. *Behavior Therapy,* 1974, 5:549.

Lazarus, A. A. Psychiatric problems precipitated by transcendental meditation. *Psychological Report,* 1976, 39:601–602.

Leitenberg, H. (Ed.). *Handbook of behavior modification and behavior therapy.* Englewood Cliffs, New Jersey: Prentice-Hall, 1976.

Liberman, R. P., and Raskin, D. E. Depression: A behavioral formulation. *Archives of General Psychiatry,* 1971, 24:515.

Lipinski, D., and Nelson, R. Problems in the use of naturalistic observation as a means of behavioral assessment. *Behavior Therapy,* 1974, 5:341–351.

McFall, R. M. Patterns of self-monitoring. In R. B. Stuart (Ed.), *Behavioral self-management: Strategies, techniques, and outcomes* (New York: Brunner/Mazel, 1977), pp. 196–214.

Mahoney, M. J., and Arnkoff, D. B. Cognitive and self-control therapies. In S. L. Garfield and A. E. Bergin (Eds.), *Handbook of psychotherapy and behavior change,* 2d ed. (New York: Wiley, 1978), pp. 661–689.

Mahoney, M. J., and Mahoney, K. Treatment of obesity: A clinical explanation. In B. J. Williams, S. Martin, and J. P. Foreyt (Eds.), *Obesity: Behavioral approaches to dietary management* (New York: Brunner/Mazel, 1976), pp. 30–39.

Mahoney, M. J., and Thoreson, C. E. (Eds.). *Self-control: Power to the person.* Monterey, California: Brooks/Cole, 1974.

Meichenbaum, D. *Cognitive behavior modification: An integrative approach.* New York: Plenum, 1977.

Miller, N. Learning of visceral and glandular responses. *Science,* 1969, 163: 434.

_____. Introduction: Current issues and key problems. In N. E. Miller, T. X. Barber, L. V. DiCara, J. Kamiya, D. Shapiro, and J. Stoyva (Eds.), *Biofeedback and self-control 1973* (Chicago: Aldine, 1974).

Murphy, L. B., and Moriarty, A. E. *Vulnerability, coping, and growth.* New Haven: Yale University Press, 1976.

Patel, C., and North, W.R.S. Randomized controlled trial of yoga and biofeedback in the management of hypertension. *Lancet,* 1975, 2:93–95.

Paul, G. L. Insight versus desensitization in psychotherapy. Stanford, California: Stanford University Press, 1966.

Pavlov, I. *Conditioned reflexes.* Oxford: Oxford University Press, 1927.

Pesnick, S. B., Filion, R., Fox, S., et al. Behavior modification in the treatment of obesity. *Psychosomatic Medicine,* 1971, 33:49.

Sargent, J., Walters, C., and Green, E. Psychosomatic self-regulation of migraine headaches. In L. Birk (Ed.), *Seminars in psychiatry,* 5 vols. (New York: Grune and Stratton, 1971), 5:415–428.

Sargent, J. D., Green, E. E., and Walters, E. D. The use of autonomic feedback training in a pilot study of migraine and tension headaches. *Headache,* 1972, 12:120–124.

_____. Preliminary report on the use of autogenic feedback training in the treatment of migraine and tension headaches. *Psychosomatic Medicine,* 1973, 35:129–135.

Schneiderman, N., Weiss, T., and Engel, B. Modification of psychosomatic behaviors. In O. F. Pomerleau and J. P. Brady (Eds.), *Behavioral medicine: Theory and practice* (Baltimore: Williams and Wilkins, 1979), pp. xxiii–xxiv.

Schwartz, G. L. Biofeedback in therapy: Some theoretical and practical issues. *American Psychologist,* 1973, 28:666–673.

Shapiro, A. P., Schwartz, G. E., and Ferguson, D.C.F. Behavioral methods in the treatment of hypertension. *Northeastern Medicine,* 1977, 86:626–636.

Skinner, B. F. *Science in human behavior.* New York: Macmillan, 1953.

Stoyva, J., and Budzynski, T. Cultivated low-arousal – an anti-stress response. In L. V. DiCara (Ed.), *Limbic and autonomic nervous systems research* (New York: Plenum, 1974).

Thoreson, C. E., and Mahoney, M. J. *Behavioral self-control.* New York: Holt, Rinehart and Winston, 1974.

Ullmann, L. P., and Krasner, L. (Eds.). *Case studies in behavior modification.* New York: Holt, Rinehart and Winston, 1965.

Voetglin, W. L., Lemere, P., et al. Conditioned reflex therapy of chronic alcoholism. *Quarterly Journal of Studies of Alcohol,* 1942, 2:505.

Weisman, A. D., and Worden, J. W. Psychosocial analysis of cancer deaths. *Omega: Journal of Death and Dying,* 1975, 6:61–75.

Wickramasekera, I. The application of verbal instruction and EMG feedback training to the management of tension headache – preliminary observations. *Headache,* 1973, 13:74–76.

Wiley, Loy. How can you improve patient compliance? *Nursing,* 1978, 8:40–47.

Williams, R. B., and Gentry, W. D. *Behavioral approaches to medical treatment.* Cambridge, Massachusetts: Ballinger, 1977.

Wolpe, J. *Psychotherapy by reciprocal inhibition.* Stanford, California: Stanford University Press, 1958.

Wolpe, J., and Lang, P. J. A fear survey schedule for use in behavior therapy. *Behavior Research and Theory,* 1964, 2:27–30.

Wooley, S. C. Physiologic versus cognitive factors in short-term food regulation in the obese and non-obese. *Psychosomatic Medicine,* 1972, 34:62–68.

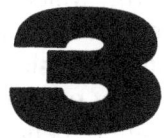

BEHAVIORAL INTERVENTION

Whatever the particular disorder, behavioral intervention requires thinking about it in behavioristic terms. Assessment of behavior throughout the treatment process is essential; this assessment should include the ways in which a physical disorder manifests itself, the situations that reinforce the symptoms, and the limitations of treatment, given the original presenting problem. In this chapter descriptions of assessment and treatment procedures for six medical disorders will be presented.

There are three steps in the intervention process: behavioral analysis, treatment, and follow-up. Behavioral analysis, or assessment, consists of the identification of carefully defined target behaviors. Information obtained from the assessment provides an understanding of the patient's assets and liabilities, suggests additional ways to observe and rate behavior, and shows how physical, psychological, and social data may be used.

The interview is the most common method of behavioral assessment (Keefe, 1975). It may be unstructured, so that the patient is encouraged to talk freely about the subject of his choice, or it may be structured around a specific item or subject. A comprehensive behavioral history is obtained; the history details maladaptive learning that may underlie the problem and the significant reinforcers of these learned habits. The target behavior is defined by encouraging the patient to communicate his experience of pain in a precise way. The health care professional must pinpoint observable behaviors that the patient can easily monitor. An evaluation of the antecedents and consequences of the behavior in question is necessary; it is best achieved by asking the patient to describe a typical day, from getting up in the morning to going to bed at night. Observation of behavior during the interview facilitates assessment of the patient's real concerns, which may differ from the initial presenting problem. The interviewer should note the patient's mannerisms, verbal styles, and any overt signs of anxiety and tension. The interviewer is in an excellent position to assess the role of verbal and nonverbal reinforcement of behavior. The therapist is important to the behavior change process despite the common misconception that he is irrelevant to such change.

Tests, questionnaires, and inventories are another aspect of behavioral analysis. Traditional psychological tests give data that may facilitate treatment planning; for example, a brain-injured person cannot reliably practice relaxation techniques. Problem-oriented questionnaires expedite the collection of data about a specific problem or target behavior. An example of such an instrument is the Fear Survey Schedule (Wolpe and Lang, 1964), which lists items that produce anxiety. The health care worker can use the patient's fear responses to the stimuli on the test in planning treatment. Monitoring by the patient himself of the behavior in question helps him to perceive the target behavior, identify its consequences and antecedents, and facilitate its modification, but direct observation of the patient in the naturalistic setting is the basic tool of behavioral assessment (Azrin, Holz, and Goldiamond, 1961; Lipinski and Nelson, 1974). Naturalistic observation – observation of the patient in his natural setting – often provides relevant information that has not been reported by the patient, and it allows the observer to assess directly environmental factors that may control or affect the target response. Observation may occur in the hospital or the home. In contrast, laboratory observation allows the practitioner to make a strong, reliable statement about the relationship between the physiological response and the environment. Blood pressure, heart rate, respiration, and electroencephalogram (EEG) can be evaluated as responses to controlled stimuli of varying strengths. Obtaining a baseline response level helps to identify precisely the subsequent changes in behavior and to assess the effectiveness of maintenance strategies.

Behavioral intervention requires extensive initial evaluation from which the second phase, treatment, flows. The term "treatment" implies that some procedures are performed on the patient. In fact, the foundation of behavioral intervention is the inclusion of the patient as a partner in his own treatment. The health care professional remains a consultant rather than a provider of direct treatment. The initial assessment is thus essential, as patients must be selected who are able to undergo behavioral intervention after an initial training period. The consultant is responsible for educating other members of the health care team about an appropriate referral, preparation of the patient for intervention, and coordination of treatment by team members.

The final phase of the intervention process, follow-up, is extremely important to maintain good results and to document the effectiveness of behavioral techniques. Near the end of treatment, sessions should gradually be spaced further apart so that the patient takes increasing responsibility for his own treatment. It is important to assess his ability to assume responsibility for behavior change without the direct contact of the therapist. Occasional "booster" treatment sessions—sessions after treatment formally stops—are often recommended to ensure that the behavior change remains.

The process of behavioral change is discussed for specific disorders—insomnia, hypertension, alcoholism, obesity, headache, and pain—in the rest of this chapter. A description of intervention and a synopsis of the relevant research is provided for each disorder; for further information see the extensive bibliography.

INSOMNIA

The term "insomnia" applies collectively to a variety of disturbances resulting in the inability to get adequate sleep. They include difficulty falling asleep and staying asleep and early morning waking (Karacan and Williams, 1971). Survey data estimate that 17–25 percent of the adult population has complained of insomnia and that 45 percent of this population has experienced insomnia as a result of psychological upset. More commonly, insomnia is associated with anxiety and depression. However, there are primary sleep disorders that may initially be described as insomnia—for example, sleep apnea (episodic cessation of respiration during sleep) and nocturnal myoclonus (periodic extensor movement of limbs associated with arousal from sleep). In addition, insomnia can accompany many medical problems, including cardiovascular disorders, alcoholism, endocrine imbalance, and neurological illness. The health care professional must be alert to the presence of insomnia and knowledgeable about treatment and management issues. It is essential to avoid the routine assumption that insomnia is "always psychological." Patients whose chief complaint is insomnia should undergo a complete evaluation, including medical review, before such arbitrary conclusions about the etiology of the insomnia are reached. As my focus is on behavioral intervention, I shall review the problem of insomnia caused by psychological difficulty, specifically, stress and tension, which is most amenable to a behavioral treatment approach. There is no evidence to suggest that behavioral intervention can directly affect a primary insomnia, such as sleep apnea.

Counseling may be helpful as an adjunct technique facilitating emotional expression of concerns that characteristically remain suppressed. By itself, however, counseling is likely to require long-term contact and produce little positive result.

Hypnotic medications are the most frequent type of intervention prescribed by physicians. However, they involve serious problems (Ribordy and Denney, 1977). They increase total sleep time, but tolerance develops quickly with nightly use for five days (Kales and Kales, 1973) and they tend to lose their effectiveness by the end of two weeks. They are associated with carry-over effects – morning hangover, drowsiness, nausea, and headache. Hypnotic substances are very slowly eliminated from the body (Oswald, 1968). Nearly all hypnotics produce disturbances in fundamental sleep patterns or staging in the form of suppressing stages Rem (the stage of sleep in which dreaming is generally reported) and 3–4 (the deep restorative stages of sleep that cause people to feel rested and refreshed on waking) sleep (Karacan and Williams, 1971; Kales and Kales, 1973). Stage 4 has a restorative function, and its suppression by hypnotic medication is ill advised. On withdrawal of medication, a sudden increase in Rem occurs, resulting in a worsening of the insomnia, severe nightmares, and dissatisfaction with the drug (Kales and Kales, 1973). These symptoms can occur after only three consecutive nights of use and may last up to several months (Kales and Berger, 1970; Oswald, 1968). As many insomniacs are already anxious and depressed, hypnotic medication may make the problem worse.

Numerous studies have distinguished between good and poor sleepers. Hauri (1970) noted that people who sleep well feel less moody, are less physically tired, and experience less fatigue. Too much sleep – more than nine hours – may also lead to a deterioration in mood and physical state. It is essential to differentiate between people who truly sleep poorly and those who report poor sleep but who manifest adequate sleep in the laboratory. Monroe (1967) used

EEG criteria to separate good from poor sleepers. Good sleepers reported a sleep latency of a few minutes; poor sleepers required up to one hour before sleep. But nocturnal awakenings were much more frequent among the insomniac group.

Misconceptions about sleep latency and length are important because hypnotics are routinely prescribed on the basis of the patient's subjective complaint. Borkovec (1979) pointed out the "need to acknowledge the heterogeneity of insomnia and specify the differences between objective insomnias as confirmed by EEG data and the subjective insomnias without confirmatory EEG data." His data also show that the patient's complaint of disturbed sleep is usually reliable, although the patient is likely not to be entirely accurate in estimating the degree of insomnia. Subjective complaints of insomnia were found to be poor predictors of objective EEG findings. The sleep laboratory is invaluable in distinguishing between subjective and objective insomnias. People complaining of insomnia are very different, and their differences must be assessed carefully as a part of treatment planning. A person's perception of how much sleep he needs is based on previous experiences and feelings. A tension-free state improves sleep; anxiety both lengthens sleep latency and increases the number of awakenings during the night. Activities like exercise and study near sleep time heighten arousal and may cause sleep-onset insomnia. Stress routinely leads to a decrease in delta (stage 3–4) sleep. One might think that increasing one's sleeptime would cause an increase in delta sleep and hence maximize one's sense of restoration and good feeling, but behavioral intervention designed to reduce the original stress is more worthwhile.

Medication is frequently used to decrease stress and make it easier for patients to fall asleep. It follows that patients tend to attribute good sleep to the medication. As a result anticipation of the withdrawal of the medication may precipitate fear, which is likely to compound the insomnia. The apprehension is confirmed by the insomnia that does occur with the withdrawal of medication.

Because so many difficulties are encountered with hypnotic medication, behavioral interventions should be considered carefully. Although they vary in method, all are based on the notion that insomnia is a result of heightened physiological arousal before and during sleep. Studies of systematic desensitization for the treatment of insomnia (Borkovec, Steinmark, and Nau, 1973; Evans and Bond, 1969; Geer and Katkin, 1966) indicate that it is effective. Only one study, however, had a control group, and as will be shown shortly, the consensus is that systematic desensitization may be no more effective than simple relaxation.

A second behavioral technique consists of training people to achieve a state of relaxation in order to facilitate sleep. Progressive relaxation, the systematic tensing and relaxing of major muscle groups in the body (Jacobson, 1938), is the most common technique. It has been extensively investigated (Borkovec and Fowles, 1973; Budzynski, 1978; Budzynski, Stoyva, and Adler, 1970; Haynes et al., 1975; Nicassio and Bootzin, 1974; Peper, 1973; Raskin, Johnson, and Rondertvedt, 1973), and researchers agree that general relaxation procedures are effective in alleviating insomnia. Premature enthusiasm, however, should be discouraged. Methodological problems in some of these studies—for example, physiological measures before and after training are not routinely collected in the sleep setting—mean that an accurate assessment of relaxation cannot be made.

Two exemplary studies of relaxation suggest that what makes relaxation effective is the systematic release of tension throughout various muscle groups in the body. Borkovec and Fowles (1973) studied female college students with subjective complaints of insomnia. They were randomly assigned to one of four groups: self training in relaxation, therapist-administered relaxation training, hypnosis-induced relaxation, and a control group (no treatment). Each subject underwent three therapy sessions lasting one hour and was told to practice relaxation just before bedtime. Significant improvement in the insomnia was noted in all three of the experimental groups; no improvement was noted in the control group. Steinmark and Borkovec (1973) randomly assigned forty-eight insomniac students to one of four experimental treatments: relaxation training, relaxation training together with desensitization to sleep, placebo, and no treatment. All experimental subjects experienced a significant improvement in sleep; in contrast, the control subjects did not. Relaxation with or without desensitization was especially helpful.

Benson (1975) compared the effectiveness of biofeedback training aimed at reducing the tension in the frontalis muscle, theta feedback, and a combination of frontalis and theta feedback in decreasing sleep-onset insomnia. The experimental subjects and eight normal controls manifested improved sleep. The insomnia subjects still required 30–86 minutes to fall asleep, although this sleep latency was significantly better than the baseline. The investigation concluded that self-monitoring by recording nightly sleep latencies may be more effective than biofeedback training in alleviating problems of insomnia.

There has been increasing interest in the relevance of classical conditioning to the behavioral treatment of insomnia (Bootzin, 1972; Evans and Bond, 1969; Poser, Fenton, and Scotton, 1965). One is routinely able to sleep because the correct environmental cues for sleep are present. The process of achieving the proper cues is called stimulus control (Bootzin, 1972). Sleep improves with control of these cues. The rationale for using stimulus control techniques is that bed and bedtime are often cues for behaviors that are incompatible with falling asleep. For example, students who studied for exams in bed are apt to have difficulty falling asleep because the concentration, activity, and perhaps anxiety required for studying are incompatible with sleep. For insomniacs, behavioral treatment can consist of helping the patient to learn to separate cues for falling asleep from cues signaling other "awake" activities. To this end, stimulus control procedures (Bootzin, 1973) are suggested. The following instructions involve stimulus control:

1. Use bed only for sleeping and for sexual activity.
2. Lie down in bed only if you intend to sleep.
3. If unable to fall asleep in ten minutes, get up and go into another room and become involved in a relaxing activity. Stay up for as long a time as desired, and then return to bed and try to sleep. If you remain awake for more than ten minutes, return to the other room to relax. Repeat as often as necessary.
4. Maintain regular bedtime and waking hours during the week and on weekends.
5. Avoid napping or resting in bed during the daytime. Do not rest in bed at night unless you intend to fall asleep.

Work by Bootzin (1973) demonstrated that the technique of stimulus control is significantly more effective than relaxation training in improving sleep. Measures examined were sleep latency, number of hours slept, mood before and after sleep, and feelings on awakening in the morning.

There have been numerous studies of the merit of behavioral

treatment for insomnia, but they are marked by two major shortcomings: (1) inadequate or inconsistent measurement of insomnia, and (2) restrictions on the samples of insomniac patients included for study (Ribordy and Denney, 1977). With regard to the first issue, objective data is desirable, but it is rarely obtained. Rather, the majority of studies use self-reports of sleep behaviors, such as sleep latency and number of wakings during the night, to demonstrate the effectiveness of treatment. It is conceivable that subjects might respond to the demand characteristics of the situation and fake bad sleep. Laboratory investigation is essential to determine the baseline level of sleep and level of improvement following treatment. It is also important that subjects be unaware of the exact nature and purpose of the study, so that they will be less likely to misrepresent their true sleeping behavior. The credibility and applicability of the data obtained increase significantly if subjective self-reports are minimized or eliminated. A combination of direct behavioral observation and physiological measures is probably the most appropriate means of assessing insomniac behavior.

With regard to the second issue, the criteria for selection of insomniacs are commonly those of Borkovec (Borkovec, Steinmark, and Nau, 1973), that is, (1) insomnia for six months or more; (2) sleep latency of thirty minutes or more; and (3) no current use of drug treatment. It is clear that differences in the effectiveness of treatment, behavioral or other, demonstrated in many studies are a function of the reported severity of the insomnia and its specific type. Behavioral research with insomnia most frequently deals with severe insomniacs who have not responded to other types of treatment. Insomniacs generally start to worry excessively about falling asleep when they expend much effort to do so. They tend to feel out of control; they are concerned that resulting daytime fatigue will interfere with their lives and fear that the insomnia may be symptomatic of severe underlying emotional disturbance. These worries, unfortunately, become associated with bedtime and interfere further with falling asleep. It is important for researchers to consider these aspects of insomnia when setting up experimental protocols so as to define the population under study as precisely as possible and clarify measurement techniques.

Insomnia is a fertile area for study. Research is necessary to clarify the effect of stimulus control on sleep. The distinction must be made between mild, moderate, and severe insomnia when undertaking research on etiology and factors that maintain the symptom. We need to develop precise specifications of behavioral and physiological measures of insomnia. Follow-up is essential to allow formulation of suitable behavioral intervention and for evaluation of the insomnia before and after treatment.

HYPERTENSION

Hypertension is a major health problem today. Although it is estimated that 15–20 percent of the adult population has hypertensive illness, it often remains undiagnosed and untreated. Compliance with hypertensive treatment programs is notoriously poor, so that treatment is frequently sporadic and inadequate. Mild or borderline hypertensive patients are often not followed consistently for sustained periods. Yet, the potential severe problems resulting from hypertension are many: There is an increased rate of death from myocardial infarction, congestive heart failure, stroke, and renal difficulty. Many physicians are reluctant to prescribe drugs for patients with slightly elevated blood pressure because of the side effects of antihypertensive medication.

The view that drugs are the best form of treatment for short-term management of hypertension is particularly true because of the generally poor rate of compliance noted for this disorder with long-term drug management. Thus, biobehavioral intervention, in which relaxation training following an initial trial of drug therapy, is currently popular. Biofeedback is also an effective treatment approach. There occurs in biofeedback a translation of visceral and neural responses into a sensory analogue which is provided to the individual about his own physiological responses (Shapiro, Schwartz, and Benson, 1974). The biofeedback equipment provides information about blood pressure and feeds it back to the patient. Knowledge of success or of having produced a "good behavior" is usually sufficient to help him learn control over the visceral response of blood pressure. (For a complete account of precisely how systolic and diastolic blood pressures are recorded, the biofeedback process, and the quality of reinforcements awarded for small changes in these parameters, see Tursky, Shapiro, and Schwartz [1972].)

Many studies attest to the utility of biofeedback in treating hypertension. After reviewing the literature, Blanchard and Young (1973) asserted that biofeedback can significantly lower both systolic and diastolic blood pressures of patients with hypertension. They also criticized the existing research for documenting only small changes in blood pressure after treatment, for minimal follow-up data, and for a lack of generalizability of findings. Biofeedback initially was conducted exclusively by professionals in their offices. Of late, however, biofeedback equipment has been manufactured that can be used in the home. The result has been a flurry of studies employing a combination of office- and home-based biofeedback training. An early problem with biofeedback was the generalization of training from the office to the naturalistic setting; the current availability of portable biofeedback equipment has minimized this concern.

Kleinman, Goldman, Snow, and Kozol (1976) showed that biofeedback could be generalized from the laboratory to the home for long-term maintenance of lowered blood pressure: When patients took their own blood pressure during a follow-up period for an experimental study of the effects of biofeedback on hypertension, they were able to maintain lowered blood pressures for four months. Krist and Engel (1975) demonstrated that patients had learned to control systolic blood pressure in three weeks of biofeedback training with a therapist and three months of home practice. Follow-up evaluation showed that the improvement lasted for at least three months. Benson (1975) obtained a stable baseline of systolic blood pressure with seven patients. During biofeedback training, reinforcement was given for blood pressure reduction, and training continued until five consecutive sessions passed without change in blood pressure. Unfortunately, no control subjects were included, and biofeedback training was never discontinued to see if blood pressure returned to the pretraining level or remained stable. Other studies too numerous to list describe the lowering of systolic blood pressure in patients with essential hypertension through biofeedback training.

There are also many studies of the effects of biofeedback on diastolic blood pressure. Miller (1969) offered biofeedback for forty-five-minute sessions five days a week for ten weeks to hypertensive in-patients to reduce diastolic blood pressure. The treatment was effective, and the experimental subjects who were taking substantial antihypertensive medication before the study were able to discontinue their medication. With periodic follow-up biofeedback, blood pressure readings remained low, even though the subjects had been discharged from the hospital and had returned to stressful environments. Although factors other than biofeedback might have caused or contributed to the improvement, Miller concluded that biofeedback had a significant treatment effect and that its potential role in teaching hypertensives to control blood pressure cannot be ignored. Another group of investigators (Frankel et al., 1978) described a sixteen-week trial of an approach that combined biofeedback and relaxation for the treatment of hypertension. Twenty-two hypertensive patients were randomly assigned to one of three groups: (1) diastolic blood pressure biofeedback and relaxation training, (2) five-hour blood pressure biofeedback, and (3) no intervention. Changes in blood pressure monitored outside the laboratory were minimal, and the five-hour and active biofeedback training produced similar, insignificant fluctuations in the readings. These data clearly lend no support to the hypothesis that these behavioral techniques are useful in the treatment of hypertension.

Studies conducted before 1974 suffered from weak methodology (Blanchard and Young, 1973; Schwartz and Shapiro, 1973). Later work is likely to be more valid, with the inclusion of adequate baseline data, control subjects, and satisfactory follow-up measures. But studies still vary significantly with respect to the number of training sessions, the extent of home training, and the prescribed use of relaxation, both as part of and separate from biofeedback. With the exception of Kleinman, Goldman, Snow, and Kozol (1976), investigators have not readily considered the issue of generalizability of a successful response (i.e., a significant decrease in blood pressure) from the laboratory to the naturalistic setting or to daily stressful situations. Attention to this issue is particularly important because hypertensive patients are frequently not motivated to monitor their blood pressure or comply with the prescribed medication regimen. Behavioral intervention, requiring significant time and motivation, may be more a helpful adjunct to drug therapy than a treatment in its own right.

Many studies of behavioral intervention with hypertension have utilized both biofeedback and relaxation training. The question arises whether it is more economic to teach relaxation by itself or to include it as a central feature of the more elaborate biofeedback training procedure. In addition, the precise role played by relaxation in reducing blood pressure or in facilitating the biofeedback process has not been elaborated. Relaxation and biofeedback training are notably different. The former consists of a self-induced, nonpharmacological, altered state of consciousness that can inhibit or reduce hypertension. No equipment is necessary, and fewer therapist-patient contacts are required. In contrast, biofeedback induces relaxation through monotonous, repeated stimulation. There is a shift away from the logical, internally oriented thought of relaxation training toward passivity. Blood pressure reduction is achieved by an alteration of emotional response as it is manifested physiologically.

The bulk of the evidence suggests that relaxation can significantly lower blood pressure in patients with essential hypertension. In general, investigations of relaxation and hypertension consistently employ control groups (Deabler, Fidel, and Dillenkoffer, 1973; Patel and North, 1975; Stone and DeLeo, 1976). Daily home practice of relaxation is an important variable. Studies demonstrate that subjects can reduce blood pressure significantly by daily home practice of progressive muscular relaxation (Brady, Luborsky, and Kron, 1974). A subjective sense of improvement on this variable has been rated by subjects in studies by Deabler, Fidel, and Dillenkoffer (1973). More research is needed to define the aspects of relaxation that contribute most to blood pressure stabilization and to identify potential side effects of relaxation training. Benson, Beary, and Carol (1974) noted no side effects with two practice sessions with one type of relaxation, transcendental meditation (TM), but emphasized that with more frequent practice, social withdrawal and severe insomnia occurred. Lazarus (1976) reported a suicide attempt by a subject who was an ardent TM user.

In comparison to the research on biofeedback and hypertension, studies of relaxation suggest that it is far more effective in providing nonpharmacological control of hypertension outside the laboratory. Relaxation requires no equipment, and the subject practices on his own time. Reduction in blood pressure by biofeedback is transient, whereas reduction with relaxation is apt to be longer-lasting and is thus likely to increase patient compliance with medical treatment.

The major focus of this section has been on behavioral intervention, but I should say a word about psychotherapy and counseling. No sound experimental evidence supports the contention that psychotherapy by itself reduces blood pressure. It is, however, viewed as an impressive adjunct to drug therapy. Psychotherapy enables the patient to recognize situations that produce anger and fear, to cope differently and respond differently to others, to express feelings appropriately, and to engage in behaviors that minimize the impact of stress situations. It is likely that compliance with medical treatment will increase as the patient experiences a sense of control.

Certainly, compliance with the prescribed medical regimen is a problem for hypertensive patients. Reasons commonly given for noncompliance include "I forgot to take my medication to work," "Medication makes me sick," and "I can't." Thus, a complete assessment of the patient's current status is required, including identification of the presenting medical problem, psychological state, past compliance behavior, and general mode of functioning. Specific objectives to be met during the interaction with the physician include a clear understanding of the patient's most important goal, agreement with the goals of intervention and their order of importance, and explanation by the physician of all drug effects, both adverse and positive, to ensure understanding by the patient. Distribution of educational material written at a level the patient can understand is an extremely important function of the interview. It is essential that patients learn how to help themselves, a task best accomplished through the use of pamphlets and continuous nursing attention. Regimens that require immediate and significant changes in lifestyle should be avoided. Patients who trust the treater involved with them tend to ask questions during each contact; these patients should be encouraged to discuss the impact of hypertension on their lifestyle. The health care professional should take care to allow his patients to reach conclusions independently that he has reached much earlier. An authority will not foster compliance by telling a patient exactly what to do – orders tend to alienate patients. Repeatedly giving consistent information about hypertension reinforces medication instructions and helps patients set up a regular drug-taking schedule. Working with the patient to set new priorities and develop appropriate ways to evaluate the result of medical intervention are two essential foci of intervention. But the most important objective is to detect noncompliance behaviors and correct them. To do so, the health care professional must understand whether noncompliance is caused by the patient's dissatisfaction with drug therapy or the staff or whether it indicates an underlying frustration or pessimism about the outcome of treatment.

Group treatment has been extremely helpful in producing compliance with hypertensive patients. A study by Nessman, Carnahan, and Nugent (1980) assessed compliance behavior in fifty-two previously noncompliant hypertensive patients. The subjects were randomly assigned to either a patient-run hypertension group (experimental) or a nurse-operated hypertension clinic (control). The experimental subjects were required to monitor their own blood pressure and to concentrate on self-help procedures. The control subjects listened to tapes on the management of hypertension and relied on a nurse to monitor blood pressure and adjust medication accordingly. Both groups met once a week for eight weeks. Measures of blood pressure immediately after the group treatment and subsequently at two- and six-month intervals indicated a significant decrease for the experimental patients. They had lower diastolic blood pressure, used less medication, and had better group attendance records than the control patients. These findings suggest that patient-managed groups may be more effective than traditional groups in the treatment of hypertension. Two other studies have utilized groups led by paramedics and nursing personnel. Klumbies and Eberhart (1966) reported positive findings, but they did not include a control group and they offered no information on the frequency or timing of the blood pressure recordings. Byassee, Farr, and Meyer (1976) found that significant decrease in blood pressure occurred with progressive muscular relaxation but that this gain was not maintained in follow-up evaluation.

Patient-managed groups increase the members' sense of control. Patients are able to make their own decisions. Involving patients actively in their own care facilitates behavior change and increases potential for compliance. Patients who perceive alterations in their behavior as a consequence of personal, conscious decisions are apt to experience the change as permanent; self-attributed behavior change clearly promotes compliance.

More research in this area—both new research and replication of old data—is needed to clarify the interaction among numerous subject variables and the effectiveness of relaxation training in controlling hypertension (Byassee, Farr, and Meyer, 1976; Elder and Eustis, 1975; Miall, 1971). Current data suggest that relaxation training is as effective as biofeedback in lowering blood pressure. As relaxation is generally less costly and takes less time, it is the preferable intervention. The question arises as to the generalizability of biofeedback training and the timing of the improvement noted if such generalization does in fact occur. While some data indicate that biofeedback can provide reduction in blood pressure for several months, no follow-up data show maintenance of this reduction or continuous gradual improvement over a longer period of time. Generally, investigations of behavioral intervention with hypertension have used too few subjects and too many conditioning tests to obtain statistical and apparent clinical significance of the treatment in question. In addition, many variables—length of biofeedback or relaxation training, use of follow-up, and criteria for improvement—differ so greatly among studies that the effectiveness of these techniques cannot be reliably measured (Blanchard and Young, 1973).

Future research must be strictly controlled. Each subject's physiology and psychology, as well as numerous situational and diurnal variables, must be considered to assess the interaction among them and their impact upon a behaviorally oriented approach for hypertension. Hypertension reported by patients must be objectively documented and evaluated completely throughout each study. Organ tissue damage should be determined. In view of the greater incidence of hypertension in males and blacks than in females and whites, both sex and race variables must be controlled in an experimental protocol. Ideally, patients should enter the study without having been on medication, but if drug therapy was ongoing, it should not be altered or discontinued during experimental treatment. For those with a history of medication, compliance behavior with the medication regimen must be evaluated.

Ideally, experimental and control subjects should be matched for initial blood pressure, duration of hypertension, medication usage, age, sex, and race; then the only difference between the two groups would be the presence or absence of the behavioral intervention. The importance of including a control group has been underscored by several studies: Control subjects themselves may manifest a dramatic reduction in blood pressure (Patel and North, 1975); placebo antihypertensive effects can cause a false positive in blood pressure reduction; blood pressures may decline with time alone (Grenfell, Briggs, and Holland, 1962); and merely instructing patients to lower their blood pressure can produce significant reductions (Shapiro, Redmond, and McDonald, 1975).

Stable baseline readings of blood pressure before treatment begins should be taken by someone blind to the nature of the intervention. Researchers should also record carefully those blood pressures measured at times unassociated with biofeedback and relaxation training. This is because blood pressure readings are notoriously labile in the office setting, which may itself precipitate anxiety. Treatments should be standardized: Biofeedback methodology is well defined, but relaxation techniques are varied and not easily replicated. Shapiro, Tursky, and Schwartz (1970) refer to the well-documented role of support and psychotherapy in the treatment of hypertension. This includes even the initial interaction between the patient and the health care professional before the start of formal behavioral intervention. They stress the need to identify and control these variables. Compliance with the practice and performance regimen must be assessed. And finally, the need for follow-up cannot be overemphasized. Only assessment over a sustained period will enable researchers to address such issues as the utility of postponing pharmacological therapy and the potential prevention of hypertension with behavioral intervention.

ALCOHOLISM

Alcoholism is the most serious public health problem today. The mortality rate is high, and accidental deaths associated with alcohol abuse and deaths resulting from alcohol-related medical problems, including cirrhosis of the liver, cardiovascular illness, and carcinoma (Berg, 1976; Schmidt and Popham, 1975), are on the upswing. Alcoholism is described in behavioral terms—that is, the frequency, rate, and amount of alcohol consumption and accompanying behaviors are some of the factors determining the stage of alcoholism. Alcoholism is currently termed a medical illness because it has numerous physiological manifestations and appears to be beyond the patient's voluntary control. However, both personality and behavioral factors play a strong role in precipitating and maintaining alcoholism and in the treatment process. The present discussion will focus on these issues.

Psychodynamic theory holds that there is a relationship between certain personality traits that are apparent in childhood and the development of alcoholism later in life. Generally, however, this hypothesis has not been supported; no personality traits or types have been found to be valid predictors of alcoholism (Armstrong, 1959; Southerland, Schroeder, and Tordella, 1950; Syme, 1957). In contrast to the psychodynamic approach, behavioral researchers view alcoholism as an acquired behavior. In the behavioral approach there are three hypotheses pertaining to alcohol abuse. The first is the tension-reduction hypothesis, that is, the theory that alcohol use helps decrease anxiety and that this decrease in anxiety is, in turn, adaptive for the individual. This theory has received no empirical support. The second hypothesis is that the environment rather than the physiological effects of alcohol is responsible for precipitating and maintaining alcohol abuse. According to this view, peer group pressures force people to conform to the norm of drinking (Jessor and Jessor, 1975). And, finally, the social learning hypothesis suggests that alcoholism is a function of classical and operant conditioning.

The epidemiological approach tells us that there are three levels of intervention to consider. Primary prevention focuses on the removal of the causes of an illness to prevent its occurrence. As the etiology of alcoholism has not yet been elucidated, it is inappropriate to dwell on this area. I should mention, however, that when primary prevention programs (e.g., upgrading the legal drinking age) have been set up, studies of their effectiveness have been inconclusive. Secondary prevention refers to the early identification and treatment of alcoholism. High-risk populations, such as people arrested for drunken driving, families of alcoholics, delinquents, and workers with a high absentee rate, are the focus of secondary prevention. An educational format—referring these sorts of people to established alcoholic treatment facilities—is the preferred approach to reducing the risk. Tertiary prevention—treatment of alcoholism once it occurs and is apparent to both the patient and others—has been most successful.

The behavioral approach to alcoholism involves a multidimensional treatment package and alternative treatment goals. All treatments that don't accomplish the prescribed goals are discarded and new ones established. Abstinence has always been the goal of alcoholism treatment programs. This goal was established in part because of the numerous medical problems associated with alcoholism and the serious implications of chronic drinking for the alcoholic's already impaired physical state. Other factors were the cravings that were thought to develop in alcoholics during intermittent episodes of sobriety and the loss of control during alcohol use (Nathan and Goldman, 1979). Abstinence is also a simple goal for both patients and observers to monitor because it is easily and clearly defined.

There has been increasing interest in the idea of helping alcoholics achieve controlled social drinking rather than abstinence. Much of this enthusiasm arises from studies that suggests that alcoholics tend to adopt social drinking patterns at some point, either spontaneously or during treatment (Miller and Caddy, 1977). However, the validity of these studies is questionable because of deficient methodology. Only small numbers of subjects were used, follow-up was inadequate, the initial diagnosis of alcoholism was unreliable, and the definition of what precisely constitutes controlled alcohol use after drinking was unclear. It is likely that support for the goal of controlled drinking springs from public dismay at the poor success rates for current treatment approaches rather than from sound research data. In reality, the success rate for alcoholic treatment programs that demand abstinence – Alcoholics Anonymous, for example – is documented, whereas the results of programs emphasizing the goal of controlled drinking remain uncertain. Current data indicate that sober alcoholics must stay abstinent in order to function (Nathan and Goldman, 1979). For those alcoholics who have been unable to learn to abstain despite extensive treatment, the goal of abstinence might realistically be altered to one of controlled drinking. Obviously, the alcoholic who controls his alcohol intake is likely to function better than one who engages in asocial, uncontrolled drinking. More research is needed to determine the relative merits of abstinence versus controlled drinking as a treatment goal, for whom each is appropriate, and under what conditions.

Excessive drinking is probably influenced by physiological and environmental cues. It also serves as positive reinforcement for certain behaviors that are specific to individuals. Thus, it is well suited to behavioral treatment, and many such interventions have been utilized. Aversive techniques were commonly used in the early years of the treatment of alcoholism. Electrical aversion – the pairing of the sight, smell, or taste of alcohol with an electric shock – has not been an effective treatment approach (Wilson, 1978a), and there are ethical concerns regarding its use. Use of medication that causes severe nausea when combined with alcohol is termed chemical aversion therapy. This approach has little merit by itself, but it is often effective as part of a treatment package that includes an active phase of individual counseling and social support sessions, followed by "booster" appointments. Similarly, systematic desensitization by itself is not a helpful treatment approach. If it is combined with individual and group counseling, and then drinking, anxiety abates temporarily. However, there is no indication of how long this will last or of the potential for decrease in or cessation of alcohol consumption (Pomerleau, Pertschuk, and Adkins, 1978).

Operant approaches have been successful in treating alcoholism.

One technique, contingency contracting, links performance of a desired behavior or elimination of aversive behavior to a reward. Contingency contracting requires a formal contract between patient and therapist that specifies the target behaviors of interest and the appropriate reinforcements. A common risk in determining reinforcements, however, is that a consequence thought to be positively reinforcing will actually be a punishment. For example, a spouse who asserts that she will leave her husband if he continues to drink may be positively reinforcing the alcoholism if the patient perceives marriage in a negative way. Contingency contracting is apt to be effective only if the patient and significant others agree on both the target behaviors and the reinforcements to be used in altering these behaviors.

Broad-spectrum behavioral approaches are most helpful in treating alcoholism. Lazarus (1965) emphasized the merit of such packages and suggested that the following interventions be included: (1) medical attention to physical problems related to excessive alcohol use; (2) aversive conditioning to decrease the frequency of abusive drinking; (3) behavioral assessment to identify the basis of the anxiety that underlies the drinking and that is also amenable to treatment with systematic desensitization; (4) assertiveness training to facilitate coping with stressful interpersonal situations; (5) behavioral rehearsal to develop more efficient skills for daily living; (6) hypnosis to counter-condition the characterological response of anxiety; and (7) marital therapy to assist the spouse in altering his or her role in the patient's alcoholism. In their 1973 study, Sobell and Sobell designed an "individualized behavior therapy" for alcoholics. This program consists of an assessment of the problem behavior, identification of possible responses to stress or pressure other than drinking, realistic evaluation of the chances that the patient will adopt each of these alternatives, and preparation for the patient to engage in the best alternative behavior at the appropriate time. For more information on behavioral intervention in alcoholism, see Sobell and Sobell (1973) for initial and outcome data, Cuddy, Addington, and Perkins (1978) for follow-up data, and Nathan and Lansky (1978) for their review of methodology and an excellent critique of the literature. Behavioral factors are clearly relevant to the etiology of alcoholism and to intervention, but the precise basis for the initiation, maintenance, acceleration, and patterns of deterioration with respect to alcoholism remain poorly understood. These areas need further research.

OBESITY

Obesity is a widespread health problem. Hazards associated with obesity are numerous. They include diabetes, muscular, skeletal, and cardiovascular disorders, kidney disease, pulmonary distress, pregnancy complications, early mortality, and socioeconomic and emotional difficulty. Obesity is a condition of excessive fat in which the number of calories consumed exceeds the body's current needs. For most people, it is unlikely that metabolic factors account for their difficulty in controlling their weight (Mahoney and Mahoney, 1976). Rather, the distinction between fat and obese individuals is attributed to differences in motivation—how much the person values weight loss and how much control he thinks he has over his behavior. Both self-control skills and patterns of eating and activity affect the tendency to be either fat or thin.

Current thinking about the etiology and treatment of obesity can be summarized in the following way: Obesity is a complex problem. Physiological, psychological, social, and situational factors and their interactions are relevant to both the etiology and the maintenance of the disorder. It is closely tied to aspects of lifestyle that require immense effort to change. In general, the obese person needs to develop positive alternatives to eating that will suppress both the motivation to eat and the actual eating response. There are four aspects of weight control: (1) the commitment to lose weight; (2) suppressing the urge to eat with a gradual decrease in eating behavior; (3) special attention to the period immediately following weight loss when relapse is likely to occur; and (4) coping with psychosocial problems likely to arise after weight loss.

Distortions in body image may underlie the individual's subjective evaluation of obesity; objective measurements of obesity are difficult. One currently accepted measure of obesity is based on the Metropolitan Life Insurance tables, which list ideal weights for men and women according to height and frame. However, the normative data start at age 25 for males and at age 18 for women, and there is no reliable basis for choosing frame size (Keys and Grande, 1973). In addition, these tables account for weight secondary to lean body mass as opposed to total body mass. This causes further distortion in the interpretation of the data.

Obese individuals do not necessarily have similar personalities. They do not routinely share personality characteristics of being externally focused or depressed (Leon and Roth, 1977). Schacter (1971) and Schacter and Rodin (1974) reported that obese people manifest heightened sensitivity to salient external cues and a high level of emotionality, but Leon and Roth (1977) presented convincing data to counter this view. For those for whom obesity is defined as a problem, there are elevations on the *Pt* and *D* scales of the Minnesota Multiphasic Personality Scale suggestive of a harsh, self-recriminative style, anxiety, and depression. The generally accepted view is that no unitary concept of obesity exists. It is important to specify precisely what is meant by obesity with respect to age of onset, pattern of development, and percentage above ideal body weight.

Some investigators assert that behavioral, psychological, and medical interventions in obesity have yielded discouraging results (Stunkard and McLaren-Hume, 1959; Suczek, 1955). They point out that weight control programs have high attrition rates, ranging from 20–80 percent. Later reports, however, suggest that behavioral approaches have a better chance of producing weight loss than do other methods (Ferster, Nurnberger, and Levitt, 1962) and emphasize the need to view overeating, including its development, maintenance, and potential for change, as a learned behavior (Ullmann and Krasner, 1965). Behavioral assessment of obesity requires specification of the problem area, collection of data on the etiology and nature of the eating, identification of eating patterns, and examination of possible solutions and alternative behaviors. The behavioral approach focuses on helping the obese patient accept the goal of positive change, examine the antecedents and consequences of weight loss behavior, and employ treatment strategies designed to meet patient's needs.

Behaviorists see obesity (exclusive of hormonal disorders) as the "result of a positive energy balance created by excessive caloric intake relative to energy expenditure" (Kolotkin, 1978:2). They focus on overeating and underexercise, which are probably overlearned habits conditioned to a variety of environmental stimuli and reinforced by immediate gratification (Stuart, 1971). The long-term consequences of overeating are weight gain and poor self-esteem; those of weight loss include improved health and appearance. Fatigue and bodily aches following the eating behavior are usually delayed, so that underexercising is likely to follow overeating. The antecedent events—physiological, psychological, or environmental—that trigger the behavior must be identified. It is important to alter the antecedent and consequent events rather than to focus on weight loss. Very gradual weight loss—one to two pounds weekly—is usual with a behavioral approach (Stuart and Davis, 1972). The long-term focus is on modification of the diet and exercise schedule; emphasis on permanent changes in habits probably underlies the higher success rate for behavioral treatment approaches for obesity than for other modalities.

The first application of behavior therapy to the treatment of obesity, reported by Ferster, Nurnberger, and Levitt (1962), had a marginal success rate. Since then, several strategies have been recommended. Stimulus control is a popular approach based on the notion that obese individuals need to bring their eating behavior under control. In this approach, it is suggested that people eat on specific prearranged occasions and set aside special eating sessions to coincide with infrequent events, such as birthdays. Thus, all eating should be done in one sitting at a specific time and should remain an activity separate from any others. Food stimuli must be kept discrete. The goal is to obtain voluntary control of eating by associating it with a specific set of environmental stimuli. Consequence control is another technique based on the role of reinforcement and punishment in maintaining or curtailing eating (Harmatz and Lepuc, 1968; Mann, 1972). The obese person understands that he can arrange the consequences of his behavior: for example, if he wants to raid the refrigerator, will candy be easily available? Prearranging the environment so that tempting foods aren't present is the emphasis in consequence control. Changing eating style—eating slowly, taking time out during meals to develop better control—helps decrease the rate and amount of food consumption. Ferster, Nurnberger, and Levitt (1962) reported an average loss of 10 pounds in ten subjects. Stuart (1967) found that eight women who underwent this program had a mean loss of 37.5 pounds in one year. Stimulus control was the primary approach but covert sensitization was also used (Cautela, 1968). In covert sensitization, the subject imagines the undesirable act of overeating and then pictures the ensuing state of nausea, so that there is an imagined association of nausea with eating. The effectiveness of covert sensitization alone has not been documented (Foreyt and Hagen, 1973; Harris, 1969).

Self-monitoring methods have been a valuable form of intervention in obesity. Data suggest that monitoring of food intake by the obese person can be effective if such monitoring occurs before the food is eaten. Recording intake after it occurs may actually cause the eating behavior to increase (Bellack, Rozensky, and Schwartz, 1974). Schachter (1971) stressed the importance of keeping food in the kitchen only, eating at restricted times, eating slowly, and pausing between mouthfuls. He reported that self-monitoring activity yields a modest decrease in eating. McReynolds, Lutz, Paulsen, and Kohrs (1976) investigated the role of stimulus control as part of a complex behavioral package that included self-reward, self-punishment, self-monitoring, and shaping, or gradually altering one's eating behavior to meet a desired goal by gradually increasing reinforcements. All techniques produced weight loss at the end of treatment, but stimulus control was superior at both three- and six-month follow-ups. The researchers concluded that many features of a traditional behavioral treatment package may not be relevant. Studies also indicate that there is no difference in weight loss between obese individuals who monitored themselves and attempted to control their eating by themselves and those obtaining reward from an external source, the therapist (Abraham and Allen, 1974). A review of the literature (Romanczyk, 1974) suggests that self-monitoring of daily calorie intake is an essential aspect of the behavioral treatment of obesity.

Cognitive methods have been used recently as part of a treatment package for obesity (Mahoney and Mahoney, 1976). Cognitive restructuring in particular teaches patients to perceive and change irrational and perfectionistic thinking that interferes with effective functioning (Beck, 1976; Ellis, 1962). Changing patients' false beliefs about their weight problems allows them to feel in better control of themselves, particularly in terms of emotionality and self-image. Formulating reasonable and flexible goals that can be put into practice is an important part of cognitive restructuring. Patients must specify how they plan to lose weight; behavior, not ideas, results in weight loss. Negative monologues that offer excuses for not sticking to a weight control program are replaced with appropriate self-evaluation statements. Problem-solving skills and increased awareness of the impact of thoughts and feelings on behavior are emphasized, and positive thinking and realistic goal-setting are encouraged. Mahoney and Mahoney (1976) reported that obese people who underwent treatment with a cognitive-behavioral, self-control approach lost significant amounts of weight.

The merit of behavioral intervention is well documented in a study by Wollersheim (1970). Following an eighteen-week period in which baseline data regarding eating patterns were collected, seventy-nine obese female college students were randomly assigned to one of the following types of treatment: social pressure and positive expectation; group behavior therapy based on learning principles and stressing the treatment of obesity; nonspecific therapy; and a control group who received no treatment. Groups met for ten sessions over a twelve-week period. Posttreatment and eight-week follow-up data indicated that the behavioral group had an early reduction in weight loss and a reduction in eating behavior. No symptom substitution occurred. This study demonstrates the effectiveness of using group therapy for obesity because of a low attrition rate. Wollersheim acknowledged that her study had a major limitation – the relatively short treatment period given the marked obesity of her subjects. Thus, many people who lost a significant amount of weight were still quite obese. In addition, she noted that whereas behavioral intervention focusing only on weight loss was initially appropriate by itself, subsequent follow-up groups focusing on social pressure and reinforcement to foster additional weight loss are helpful. Because this study obtained significant findings in a field so full of failures, replication of this research is important. Kingsley and Wilson (1978) demonstrated that group treatment yielded more weight loss during a six-month follow-up evaluation than did individual therapy. Their subjects initially acquired skills that enabled them to lose weight and then their motivation was reinforced by the group.

The role of family variables in weight loss has not been systematically evaluated. The obese person's need for praise, encouragement, and cooperation from friends must serve as reinforcement for continued involvement in treatment – but unfortunately, there is no empirical support for this statement.

Because of increasing confidence that behavioral interventions facilitate weight loss, "packages" of behavioral techniques that focus on specific behaviors related to obesity have been developed. These packages contain combinations of the following approaches: self-monitoring, therapist reinforcement, contingency contracting, reinforcement by others besides the therapist for habit change, relaxation, stimulus control, cognitive structuring, aversive conditioning, and covert sensitization. Some techniques recently included in the packages are exercise, social support, and self-reinforcement. Exercise is considered an essential part of the weight-loss process (Stuart, 1971). Unfortunately, many investigators see obesity as a disorder of eating that requires changing only that particular activity in one's lifestyle. The involvement of a cooperative spouse in the treatment of obesity is important. In specific studies (Mahoney and Mahoney, 1976), obese subjects who underwent behavioral training and had cooperative spouses lost an average of 30 pounds over a treatment period of eight and one-half months, and two-thirds of this group maintained the weight loss for a significant period. Self-reinforcement means that people reward themselves appropriately when they attain prearranged goals. This is an effective part of a treatment package; it builds self-esteem by encouraging people to feel responsible for their successes as well as their failures in a weight loss program.

Behavioral interventions for the treatment of obesity are very popular because they yield positive and objective findings that can be precisely measured. Studies investigating the effectiveness of these interventions, however, are of limited value because of methodological flaws (Wilson, 1978). Most studies do follow-up assessments only ten to fifteen weeks after weight loss. It is difficult to maintain weight loss for long periods, so that the reported superiority of behavioral intervention may be based on rapid but short-lived weight loss rather than the long-term maintenance that many researchers imply in their discussion of the data. Methods of selecting subjects for study also require attention. Many studies use college students as subjects; hence it is questionable whether the results are generalizable to other groups. Another significant problem is the frequent heterogeneity of the sample; individual differences in age, sex, and socioeconomic status, for example, are uncontrolled. These differences, rather than the intervention itself, may underlie the positive findings. For example, it has been determined that the age of onset of obesity significantly affects response to treatment (Grinker, 1973). Many studies do not have a control group, which makes any positive results inconclusive. A related frequent problem is the inclusion of a no-treatment control group. This is viewed as inadequate (Jeffrey, 1975) because it allows conclusions only about the effects of behavioral intervention versus no intervention. It is better to use a control group that undergoes nonspecific behavioral training, which would permit researchers to make statements about the utility of the specific behavioral technique employed. A final methodological problem is the selection of the dependent variable. The way in which a treatment outcome is measured varies among investigations. Simple weight change (Gormally, Buese-Moscati, Clyman, and Forbes, 1977) and percentage of body weight loss (Bellack, Rozensky, and Schwartz, 1974) are two common measures of outcome. It is better to use several measures to ensure that the data will be valid.

Mahoney (1976) underscored the need for better research in the area of behavioral intervention for obesity. He recommended that studies include accurate procedural descriptions, nontreatment control subjects, complete reports of outcome data for all subjects, adequate follow-up periods and assessment, and consideration of potential contributors to change, such as the patient's beliefs and attitudes about weight, diet, and weight loss.

Behavioral programs have been consistently found to be better than individual and group therapy in facilitating weight loss (Wilson, 1978). This conclusion, however, seems to be based on brief studies with inadequate follow-up evaluation. Although weight loss may occur, it may not be statistically significant. In addition, people respond differently to various behavioral approaches. Among groups that receive some treatment instructions, weight loss may vary as much as 75 pounds. Psychological predictors of this variability are unknown (Weiss, 1977), and physiological factors have not been adequately investigated by the behaviorists. It has not been proved that behavioral intervention can maintain weight loss. In part, this stems from the absence of long-term follow-up to assess maintenance. In addition, attrition rates are high. When monetary deposits and rewards are used as reinforcement for weight-loss behavior, the dropout rate does decrease (Abraham and Allen, 1974; Foreyt and Hagen, 1973; Hagen, Foreyt, and Durham, 1976; Manno and Marston, 1972).

Learning principles are an important part of obesity treatment (Stuart, 1967), but by themselves they are inadequate. There is a need for a "package" with a variety of techniques aimed at changing specific behaviors. Some behavioral techniques (e.g., booster sessions, cognitive techniques) have not been completely investigated; they may be valuable as part of a multifocus behavioral package. Problems that might be addressed in studies of potential combined treatment approaches include (1) the subject who does not comply with the therapist's intervention plan but who nevertheless loses weight; (2) weight loss during treatment that may be correlated only with self-report of behavior change, so that researchers will not know what caused the weight loss, and (3) the actual components of behavioral packages of treatment.

We may increase the probability that behavioral programs for the treatment of obesity will have positive outcomes (i.e., weight loss) by helping patients adopt goals of changing eating-related behaviors as appropriate. Specific goals for eating and exercise behaviors are best set through the free cooperation of the patient and therapist before intervention. The emphasis is on individual methods to control the urge to eat rather than directly on the eating behavior. A strong effort must be made to deliver intervention so as to maximize patient compliance and participation in an ongoing evaluation of the compliance and of the intervention process during intervention. And, perhaps most important, the behavioral intervention should include a program for the long-term maintenance of weight loss. Interdisciplinary collaboration among health care professionals is strongly urged so as to provide integration of the process of weight loss with personality change and maintenance of a satisfactory adjustment.

HEADACHE

The host of prescription and over-the-counter headache medications show that headaches are extremely common. Headache constitutes a major medical problem; the pain is severe, often disabling, causing substantial absences from work. In this section, discussion will focus on headache in general as well as two specific types of headaches, muscle-tension and migraine. Muscle-tension headache presents as a steady symmetrical ache in the occipital or bitemporal area. It is frequently described as a tight, bandlike pressure around the head (Williams and Gentry, 1977). Migraines are vascular headaches and consist of a steady, throbbing pain, initially unilateral and later more diffuse, that lasts up to four days. They are frequently accompanied by nausea and vomiting, although these symptoms may also appear as part of a prodromal syndrome (Diamond and Baltes, 1973; Williams and Gentry, 1977). Although migraine patients have a higher degree of muscle tension in the frontalis (forehead) muscle than do muscle-tension headache patients, the presence of frontalis tension cannot be used to distinguish between the two types (Philips, 1978). There is only a weak association between level of frontalis muscle-tension as measured by the electromyogram (EMG) and the intensity and frequency of headache, and the relationship that does exist is very complex. The distinction between muscle-tension and migraine headache is frequently blurry, and diagnosis by exclusion becomes necessary: that is, a headache in the absence of symptoms characteristic of migraines, such as nausea and photic phenomena, is likely to be termed muscle-tension.

Sensory input, arterial constriction and dilation, and muscular contraction are considered important in the etiology of headache, but there is also substantial concern for psychological factors involved in the initiation or maintenance of headache symptoms (D'Alessio, 1972). Certain personality traits are characteristic of headache sufferers; these are relevant to treatment decisions and long-term management of these patients. Psychological variables that contribute to the onset of headache or accompany pain are frequently noted by the health care professional but, unfortunately, do not receive adequate attention.

Headache patients have been described in the psychoanalytic literature as intelligent but emotionally unstable (Cushman, Gray, and Moore, 1943), overcontrolled, perfectionistic, and ambitious (Knopf, 1935), and unable to express anger except by turning it inward (Fromm-Reichmann, 1937). A more recent investigation by Beck (1976) concurs with these views. However, there are no reports of controlled studies using matched subjects to confirm or reject these descriptions. The notion of a "headache personality" is no longer popular. Philips (1977) found that a random sample of headache sufferers were no more neurotic or psychotic than the general population. Subdivision of the sample into migraine and muscle-tension headache groups also revealed no differences on measures of neuroticism and psychoticism. Diamond and Baltes (1973) felt that migraine patients suffer from an underlying depressive illness and emphasized the need to assess personality fully before formulating a treatment plan. It should also be recognized, however, that many apparent psychological difficulties reported by headache patients—inability to function, disruption of one's life, and such emotional manifestations as resentment and irritability—may result from the chronic experience of pain.

Behavioral approaches are well-suited to the treatment of headache. The most frequently used interventions are biofeedback (frontal EMG feedback) and relaxation training, although self-monitoring, self-management, and cognitive approaches have also been used. A brief literature review will be presented to demonstrate the effectiveness of some types of behavioral intervention in the treatment of muscle-tension and migraine headache.

Data suggest that a variety of behavioral interventions can reduce the frequency, intensity, and duration of muscle-tension headache. Most studies focus on the patient's response to stressors rather than the reduction of those stressors (Mitchell and White, 1976) that may have originally caused the headache. Because tension headache results from sustained contractions of the neck and scalp musculature, reduction of tension in these areas may eliminate the headaches (Sainsbury and Gibson, 1954). Many reports attest to the success of this procedure. In these studies subjects underwent biofeedback training in which varying quality tones provided information about the extent of muscle tension. Significant decreases were noted in frontalis muscle tension (EMG) (Budzynski et al., 1970; Budzynski et al., 1973; Wickramasekera, 1972).

Studies of the effectiveness of behavioral treatment in headache management that include a matched control group are of greater value. Work by Budzynski, Stoyva, and Mullaney (1973) was the first controlled study reported in the literature. Subjects monitored the frequency and nature of their headaches for a two-week baseline period; they then participated in twice-weekly sessions for sixteen weeks in one of the following treatment conditions: frontal EMG biofeedback, pseudofeedback (feedback of a variable tone that is not correlated with frontal EMG), or no feedback. The EMG biofeedback group was able to decrease frontalis tension significantly more than either of the other two groups and to maintain that improvement for three months following intervention. Haynes, Griffin, Mooney, and Parise (1975) found that subjects who worked with a therapist in biofeedback and relaxation training reported a greater reduction in the frequency of headaches than control group subjects who practiced relaxation alone. Follow-up data at five to seven months showed that the improvement continued. Similar results were reported by Cox, Freundlich, and Meyer (1975) for a four-month follow-up period.

Budzynski (1978) obtained interesting results in a study of the effect of frontalis EMG biofeedback on muscle-tension headache: (1) During a two-week pretraining period, placebo effects were noted in 25 percent of the subjects. These effects were transient and disappeared within two weeks. (2) Subjects undergoing frontalis biofeedback training had significantly less muscle tension than did control subjects with no training. (3) Although both the frontalis EMG biofeedback and control groups practiced relaxation twice daily at home, still only the former group reported fewer headaches. (4) A significant number of subjects noted a significant decrease in the frequency of headaches with two biofeedback training sessions per week. (5) The biofeedback group used significantly fewer tranquilizers and pain medications than either the pseudofeedback or control group. (6) Subjects reported the following in the course of biofeedack training: inability to cope with headaches; awareness of muscle tension prior to onset of the headache and some ability to relax; heightened awareness of muscle tension prior to headache onset, ability to relax and abort a moderate headache; and automatic relaxation when faced with stress or the early stage of headache. Home practice with relaxation following the last biofeedback session was found to be essential to maintain the lower frequency of headaches.

A number of studies have demonstrated that a treatment package that includes both relaxation and frontalis EMG feedback leads to significantly fewer muscle-tension headaches than either a placebo feedback or no treatment and that this reduction lasted for a three-to-twelve-month follow-up period. No statistically significant difference has been noted in the effectiveness of relaxation and that of frontalis EMG feedback in treating muscle-tension headache (Chesney and Shelton, 1976; Kondo and Canter, 1977; Philips, 1977). As relaxation training requires no ongoing contact with a health care professional, no equipment, and less practice time than the biofeedback modality, relaxation is probably more cost-efficient than biofeedback. A number of studies have considered this possibility. Most included a frontalis biofeedback group, a nonbiofeedback relaxation or pseudofeedback group, and a no-treatment control group (Chesney and Shelton, 1976; Wickramasekera, 1973). Because of the differing methodologies they employed—varying screening criteria for inclusion of subjects, types and goals of feedback, lengths of training periods and instructions—it is difficult to compare them. Still, their results—no differences between biofeedback and no-treatment (Chesney and Shelton, 1976), greater reduction in headache from biofeedback as opposed to no training (Wickramasekera, 1972, 1973), and lack of difference between biofeedback and relaxation, both of which facilitated headache reduction (Cox, Freundlich, and Meyer, 1975; Haynes, Griffin, Mooney, and Parise, 1975)—support the conclusion that frontalis EMG biofeedback, alone or in combination with relaxation, decreases the frequency of headaches.

There has been extensive investigation of migraine headaches because they are often disabling as a result of severe pain and associated unpleasant somatic manifestations. Most studies have looked at the effects of a combined relaxation and biofeedback treatment program on headache frequency; few have studied biofeedback only. Friar (1974) studied migraine patients who kept logs of their headaches thirty days before and thirty days after an eight-week period during which they had biofeedback training sessions once a week. There was a significant reduction in migraine frequency after the treatment. EMG biofeedback is useful in treating migraine because it provides information about a given muscle site that permits quantifaction of the tension level observed and gradual shaping of the relaxation response. For more detailed information on the apparatus and training methods, consult Thompson and Patterson (1974).

Most studies of migraine headaches rely on hand temperature, usually recorded from the finger tip, as the main form of biofeedback. The rationale for this biofeedback approach is that the pain of migraine is a result of the dilation of cranial arteries. It is well described by Sargent, Walters, and Green (1973:418–419): "In the case of migraine which appears to be part of a stress-related syndrome, the somatic response is a dysfunction of vascular behavior in the hand which is related to intense sympathetic dysfunction. Vasoconstriction in the hands signals probable sympathetic outflow. It seems reasonable to hypothesize that autogenic feedback training for hand-warming is effective in the amelioration of migraine because patients have to 'turn off' excessive sympathetic outflow."

The hypothesis that migraine stems from heightened sympathetic activation underlies many studies that have used thermal biofeedback training. Blanchard and Young (1974) compared the effectiveness of thermal digital vasomotor training (thermal biofeedback) to that of progressive relaxation. Both treatments significantly reduced the frequency and intensity of migraine headaches. Another form of treatment for migraine is autogenic training, which was developed by J. M. Shultz (Schultz and Luthe, 1969). It consists of a combination of techniques—self-monitoring exercises, hypnosis, yoga, and relaxation training. These techniques are accompanied by a set of physiological exercises requiring passive concentration; they are designed to reduce heaviness in the extremities and to bring heart rate, pulse, and respiration to appropriate levels. Green and his associates (Green, Green, and Walters, 1970; Sargent, Green, and

Walters, 1973) reported a successful clinical outcome with autogenic feedback training (a combination of autogenic training and thermal biofeedback) for migraine headache. Other controlled research of temperature biofeedback, either alone or combined with autogenic training, has not shown that these types of intervention reduce migraine frequency (Friar, 1974; Turin and Johnson, 1976).

When the health care professional is confronted with a patient complaining of headache, he must first determine its etiology. Neurological illness and other serious organic problems must be ruled out by a physician. Once a diagnosis of muscle-tension headache or migraine is established, behavioral treatment can be considered. Behavioral intervention typically attempts to reduce psychophysiological arousal and muscle-tension levels in the musculature of the head and neck. D'Alessio (1972) noted the need to assess the role of multiple psychophysiological conflicts that might precipitate headache and of secondary gain issues. If psychological factors are relevant, psychotherapy combined with biofeedback is appropriate. There are, however, no evaluations of the effectiveness of psychotherapy with headache patients.

Most headache patients have tried many types of medication without positive result. The most commonly used is aspirin, although tranquilizers and muscle relaxants are also routinely and heavily prescribed. Drug dependence is a common problem with headache patients, in part because medication is so frequently prescribed and in part because its positive effects are only transient, so that patients may take too many pills. Patients who are taking analgesics and sedatives—Fiorinal, for example—will need to decrease medication gradually and ultimately discontinue it altogether during the course of behavioral intervention.

Concern about the side effects of chronic medication use has prompted an active search for effective nonpharmacological forms of intervention. Here behavioral strategies hold promise. The frequency and intensity of headaches vary according to psychological and environmental stress. Although this has not been definitively established, some people do seem to respond to stress with muscle contractions of the head and neck. Headache is often a result of environmental cues; for example, headaches that routinely start in social situations may lead to future avoidance of the headache-producing situation. Epstein and Abel (1977) and Friedman (1964) reported that pharmacological intervention reduced muscle tension in patients with muscle-tension headaches but that the patients still complained of headaches. Another way of treating these patients is to reduce anxiety by systematic desensitization before the start of pharmacological therapy. As patients come to feel less anxious and better able to cope without medication, drug use can be tapered off and ultimately stopped. When medication is discontinued, patients can undergo behavioral treatment to learn to ward off headaches at their onset. There is some evidence that effective biofeedback training with headache patients depends on rapport between the health care professional and the patient (Fahrion, 1977; Taub and Emurian, 1971).

Other forms of intervention have been utilized with headache patients. Placebo expectancy—anticipation by the patient of a successful outcome because of information given by the clinician—is often helpful in combination with other types of intervention. If unrealistic expectations are established, a high treatment dropout rate will occur as the expectations are not fulfilled. Clinicians should set realistic expectations. One researcher has reported a 70–80 percent "cure" rate with biofeedback training and home practice continuing for at least three months following the initial treatment (Wickramasekera, 1972). A useful review of the placebo literature can be found in Stroebel and Glueck (1973).

Another type of intervention, cognitive skills training, focuses on the modification of negative thoughts and on the uncovering of the false assumptions that may precipitate such thoughts. The goal is to achieve more realistic positive ideation. Patients should practice using positive coping statements when confronted with stress and then undergo six to eight weeks of frontalis EMG biofeedback. Talking about the stressful situation is less helpful than learning positive cognition ("I can relax and handle this situation"). Obviously it is easier to modify maladaptive thoughts if one is able to relax, so mastering relaxation skills should precede cognitive skill training. According to Borkovec (1979), cognitive skills training is less effective when the patient is anxious because of a high physiological arousal.

A treatment package consisting of biofeedback, relaxation, altered cognition, and dealing with everyday stresses is recommended. We need to identify the components of such packages and their relative effectiveness. Patients have to make a great effort to maintain their therapeutic success and the transfer of biofeedback-learned skills to the home and other outside settings. Home practice is often neglected, but patients can arrange appropriate remedies—for example, using a mechanical alarm wristwatch that buzzes every one to two hours (Budzynski, 1978). Probably the best results with headache patients occur in settings that combine biofeedback with a supplemental treatment. Although there is a lack of evidence for the efficacy of psychotherapy for headache sufferers, this approach would seem to be particularly helpful in dealing with issues of secondary gain. For example, a person may be unmotivated to learn to ease headache if its pain allows him to avoid participation in social situations. If coping skills were fostered by psychotherapy, entry into biofeedback might be a stronger possibility. A seemingly worthwhile treatment package is composed of (1) relaxation training to reduce the initial level of pain and anxiety; (2) techniques like psychotherapy and systematic desensitization to facilitate coping with situations that appear to trigger headache; and (3) attention to the reinforcement of the headache and complaint behavior by significant others. If others are indifferent to the headache and the patient is rewarded for healthy activity unrelated to the headache, the patient will complain less and additional psychological and social difficulties that might otherwise result from the pain behavior will be reduced.

In summary, the data suggest that frontalis EMG biofeedback may effectively alleviate or eliminate muscle-tension headache. The effectiveness of temperature biofeedback for migraine has yet to be demonstrated in well-controlled studies, although its utility has been documented in other work. Treatment packages that include biofeedback, relaxation, psychotherapy, and cognitive skills training can alleviate headache in the short term and maintain the successful outcome. Placebo expectancy may be helpful when used in combination with biofeedback or relaxation training. Before undergoing any intervention, however, patients should receive complete medical evaluations and psychological screening to assess their suitability for behavioral intervention.

Researchers need to deal with the following methodological problems: (1) Variables—for example, subject and therapist expectations, relationship variables, and baseline individual differences—are often not well controlled; (2) Too little is known about the ways in which individual differences affect the ability to learn visceral control and how to predict from personality and physical factors whether biofeedback treatment for headache will be successful; (3) It is not clear whether laboratory-learned biofeedback skills can be generalized to the home setting; (4) Blind retrospective studies to control for potential placebo effects are needed; (5) Control groups are not always used; (6) Samples are often very small; and (7) Some investigators tend to confuse biofeedback with other behavioral interventions and to avoid reporting the details of the treatment actually used.

Specific suggestions for improved clinical service include: (1) baseline biofeedback training for at least four weeks before treatment; (2) routine assessment of compliance with recommended home practice during the treatment and follow-up phases; (3) evaluation of the extent of secondary gain operating to reinforce the headache symptom; (4) referral of patients who can attain relief of headache from nonbiofeedback intervention to the appropriate type of treatment; (5) separation of individuals into groups based on the amount of frontalis tension as measured by EMG; and (6) logging by patients of the frequency and intensity of headaches for approximately four weeks after intervention, with additional regular follow-up evaluations in person with the clinician.

PAIN

It is popularly believed that pain is a result of illness or trauma and that it is always felt in direct proportion to the degree of injury. In fact, although pain may cause people to seek medical evaluation, it can have either psychological or organic bases. Pain can occur as a result of unknown organic pathology, so that there may be no direct relationship between tissue injury and the extent of pain perceived by the patient. Pain perception may be influenced by several variables: for example, anxiety causes a greater intensity of pain; females tend to be described as complaining more about pain as a consequence of sex stereotyping; and pain tolerance decreases with age. In addition, there are cultural differences in the experience of pain (Sternbach and Tursky, 1965).

The many attempts that have been made to define pain attest to its complexity as a concept. The following descriptions are particularly illustrative. Weisenberg (1977:1009) stated that "pain is in some respects a sensation; in other respects, it is an emotionally-motivated phenomenon that leads to escape and avoidance behavior." Sternbach (1968:12) wrote that "pain appears to be an abstraction we use to refer to different feelings which have little in common except the quality of physical hurt . . . a class of behaviors which operate to protect the organism from harm or enlist aid in effecting relief."

Pain is manifested in behavior, so that diagnostic inferences and decisions about treatment can be made. Both verbal and nonverbal cues signal the intensity, frequency, location, and quality of the pain (Sternbach, 1968). Pain is a sensory phenomenon, but its infinite behavioral manifestations help the health care professional to distinguish between acute and chronic pain. People experiencing acute pain usually consult a physician and note relief quickly with prescribed treatment. Other forms of pain, however, do not remit easily, and the recommended treatment plans (e.g., surgery, medication) may not be effective. At this point the chronic pain course starts. Level of anxiety also distinguishes acute from chronic pain: Acute pain patients experience heightened and lowered anxiety consonant with the large or small amounts of pain, whereas chronic patients feel a sustained anxiety accompanied by a sense of helplessness and frustration. If health care professionals are tempted to intimate that this kind of pain is not real and that psychotherapy is needed, the anxiety may escalate.

Pain is routinely labeled psychogenic if there is no demonstrable cause or if there is inconsistency between the reported degree of pain and measurements of physiological sensations and parameters. Pain may also be termed psychogenic when emotional factors are merely assumed to be the primary cause of pain (Merskey, 1968; Spear, 1967; Sternbach, 1974).

The disease model of pain predicts that eliminating or treating the body damage will cause the pain to disappear. The assumption underlying this model—that pathology is the source of pain—is appropriate for acute pain patients. Diagnostic procedures, however, cannot easily identify the basis of chronic pain nor can they routinely suggest a treatment plan for pain reduction. In his extensive research on pain, Fordyce (1976) considered the factors that control pain, whether real or imagined, as relevant to treatment planning. He described pain as subject to conditioning and stated that once pain is conditioned, it can also be unlearned. Pain can be reinforced by direct positive reward (e.g., attention), which in turn increases directly with pain behavior; by indirect positive reinforcement (e.g., allowing patient to miss work); and by nonreward of "well" behavior—the alternative responses to pain that are incompatible with "ill" or pain behavior (Fordyce et al., 1973). For additional readings on the management of chronic pain based on the principles of reinforcement and learning, see Bandura (1969) and Wolpe (1972).

Obviously, a complete behavioral assessment is required before an appropriate intervention can be formulated. This assessment should include the patient's relationship with family members, response of family, colleagues, and friends to his pain, and the history of the patient's use of pain medication. The assessment also ordinarily includes a personality evaluation. This addresses itself to the following issues: the current degree of emotional stress as a consequence of pain behavior, the presence of premorbid psychological difficulties, the potential for addiction or habituation to medication, the response to the withdrawal from activity and the external attention that are consequences of the pain, the significance of pain for the patient and his lifestyle, and the nature of reinforcement, if any, for normal activity. The assessment should fully consider the interaction between patient behavior and patterns of environmental reinforcement. Psychological factors play a more significant role in the experience and management of chronic pain than in the case of acute pain (Melzack and Chapman, 1973). People with high levels of anxiety, and extroverts are more intolerant of pain (Lynn and Eysenck, 1961). Psychological test data indicate that pain patients are so preoccupied with somatic problems that emotional interpersonal issues are avoided or denied altogether. Those pain patients who can acknowledge that they feel anxious and depressed because of their inability to function are likely to benefit from interventions designed to reduce pain (Pilowsky, 1968). Some chronic pain patients may utilize pain behavior to get medication or attention; secondary gain issues must be dealt with to avoid unknowingly reinforcing the pain.

Depressives complain of pain significantly more than do healthy controls but no more so than do other psychiatric groups. Pain tends to mask depression so that pain patients may not appear clinically depressed (Sternbach, 1974). Most patients are depressed because of the pain. We can think of depression as a lack of positive reinforcement. If pain causes the patient's routine activity to be curtailed, then the patient will probably have experienced a loss of usual reinforcement. The greater the pain, the more disruption in activity, and the greater the depression. Exceptions to this are situations where no loss exists, either because activity was never or rarely reinforced or because family members provide new sources of reinforcement by rewarding pain behavior. The literature suggests that pain patients, regardless of the etiological factors, are psychologically similar (Fordyce et al., 1978; Sternbach et al., 1973; Woodforde and Merskey, 1972), although chronic pain patients appear more concerned about physical symptoms and more depressed than other pain patients. Recent work by Leavitt and Garron (1979) indicates that patients who have undiagnosable back pain are more psychologically disturbed than a sample of patients with proven low back pain. The former group tends to emphasize affective and sensory components of the pain. These investigators found that "47% of the patient sample with psychological disturbance also had diagnosable organic disease and 41% of the patients without diagnosable organic disease showed no evidence of psychological disturbance." (Leavitt and Garron, 1979:194). This finding suggests that the complaint of pain and the occurrence of pain behavior do not in themselves imply the presence of psychological disturbances.

There are two treatment models for pain, respondent and operant (Fordyce, Fowler, and deLateur, 1968). The respondent treatment approach views pain as a response to an external cue for physical and muscular tension; wherever pain occurs, it stems from the tension of muscles surrounding an area where there had been an injury. Anxiety, for example, is likely to intensify one's subjective experience of pain, which in turn will increase the tension levels in nearby muscle groups. This is termed a pain-tension-pain cycle (PTP). The primary treatment modalities of the respondent model are biofeedback and relaxation in which the patient takes an active role. It should be noted that the health care professional untrained in behavioral intervention is apt to engage initially in passive treatment, for example, medication. Biofeedback, an active form of intervention, teaches the patient to monitor the level of tension in muscles surrounding the area of the body that is perceived as painful. The patient can then learn to relax whenever tension increases to the point where the pain sensation occurs.

The operant model considers the factors that initiate and maintain the pain syndrome: the relationship between pain behavior (i.e., the expression of pain) and consequences in the environment. Maladaptive pain behaviors, such as decreased activity at work and social withdrawal, constitute the focus of diagnosis and treatment. Specifically, we need to identify how these behaviors operate on the environment to cause positive or negative consequences for the patient. Pain behavior can be maintained (1) when pain elicits continued positive reinforcement, (2) when the pain experience enables the patient to avoid certain unpleasant activities, and (3) when "well behaviors" are not reinforced (Fordyce, 1976). Fordyce, Fowler, and deLateur (1968) were able to treat chronic pain patients successfully with operant techniques by changing the patterns of reinforcement: Medication for pain was distributed at specific times rather than when needed, and social reinforcement was given for improvement in functioning. In a longitudinal study including treatment and follow-up, Fordyce et al. (1973) found that an operant treatment program produced significant decreases in the amount of pain, interference of pain in daily activity, and medication, and an increase in the amount of time spent in routine activity for thirty-six patients.

The operant model is the most popular current behavioral treatment for pain. Its goals are to reduce pain and to establish and maintain well behaviors. In the pretreatment assessment of the patient, it is crucial to consider past and present treatments for pain, especially those that offer consistent positive reinforcement for maladaptive pain behaviors. Orientation for the patient and significant others is a significant part of the operant treatment program. They all need to learn how conditioning can maintain pain behavior and increase the time needed for the original injury to heal. Responsiveness to the patient is frequently demonstrated to be pain-contingent, thereby rewarding pain behavior. All should be aware of treatment goals, how they are to be obtained, and behaviors that could occur following intervention. The spouse is asked to pinpoint target behaviors with the patient, to count specific pain behaviors during twenty-minute periods so as to increase alertness to pain behaviors, to identify his or her response to the pain behaviors demonstrated by the patient, and to withdraw attention to pain behaviors, at the same time offering reinforcement of behaviors leading to specified treatment goals. It is essential to tell the patient that pain is a learned behavior and that, although his suffering is real, he is probably experiencing more pain than necessary. An important goal of treatment is to increase activity to a quota mutually agreed upon by the patient and the health care professional. The patient's tolerance for activity is not considered a factor in setting up the quota. A full explanation of the need to control the use of pain medication should be offered, and there should be a gradual tapering-off of medication if appropriate. Medication should not be abruptly changed or discontinued, and if medication is necessary, it must be taken on a time-contingent basis rather than as needed. A careful evaluation of the interaction between patient and spouse must be done. The patient and significant others must understand that the program staff will respond to well behaviors only. These include increased exercise, activity, and involvement.

Because most pain patients are using excessive amounts of medication – to the point of addiction or habituation – before intervention, a physician must determine whether the patient needs detoxification or deconditioning and must oversee medical care. Pain "cocktails" (Fordyce et al., 1978) containing gradually decreasing dosages of active pharmacological agents must be used for seven to ten weeks before medication can be withdrawn. For patients with clinical depression, antidepressant medication can be added to the pain cocktail. As noted above, the pain cocktail is taken on a time-contingent and time-limited basis.

Exercise is a response incompatible with pain behavior. When patients exercise, family members tend to express concern for the patient. As this rewards the pain behavior, family members must learn how to reinforce rather than discourage activity. Physical limits are set on an individual basis. Once exercises are selected, baseline levels are set so that the patient's early participation in the program is gradual. It is essential to build success early in the program, as the attrition rate with early failures is high. At every opportunity graphs and diagrams portraying the suitable progress of the patient should be displayed. Patients who fail to meet their quotas reestablish quotas below their baseline level. The therapist needs to record the data and continue to meet with the patient as was originally arranged. If patients repeatedly fail to meet their quotas, despite readjustments, the operant treatment approach may be inappropriate for them.

The achievement of well behaviors constitutes a primary part of the treatment program. External reinforcements that act to strengthen the pain behavior must be modified. With direct positive reinforcement, patients receive attention only when in pain, so that well behaviors are discouraged. Prescriptions for narcotics and analgesics on a p.r.n. (as needed) basis make attention in the form of medication contingent on pain; they therefore reinforce the pain. Rest is also a reinforcer; because it causes decreased activity and pain, it thus further increases the probability of additional pain as attention seeking. Time-out, or the chance for the patient to withdraw from treatment program activities, allows the patient to remove himself from stressful situations. Yet, avoidance of stress reinforces the pain behavior that initially precipitated the avoidance. Pain behavior is also reinforced by patients' modeling themselves on others who demonstrate pain behavior: Parents who readily show pain, for example, serve as effective models for their children, who will probably follow suit. Fordyce's (1976) operant conditioning program is based on this analysis of reinforcement.

The management of acute pain consists frequently of physical intervention (i.e., medication, corrective procedures). Chronic pain, however, is more difficult to treat. In-patient treatment strategies include pure and mixed behavioral approaches, which may include interventions other than reinforcement for well behaviors (e.g., group therapy, family therapy, and relaxation). The few pure operant pain treatment programs currently in existence in the United States suggest that we need to consider a mixed behavioral program. Outpatient treatment strategies include the cognitive-behavioral approach (Turk, 1978), which facilitates the modification of pain behavior and aids the patient in developing tolerance for pain, increasing activity levels, and curtailing medication. Stress innoculation (Meichenbaum and Turk, 1976) consists of practice in generating positive statements by patients about their ability to cope with stress. This technique emphasizes identification of the antecedents of pain and in vivo application of the newly learned coping mechanisms. Because the stress innoculation technique has little inherent structure and direct supervision, it encourages the patient to assume responsibility for treatment. Steger and Harper (1977) support stress innoculation, suggesting that cognitive issues have to be directly addressed if the alleviation of pain is the goal.

It is relatively easy to decrease pain behavior; it is more difficult to replace pain behaviors with well behaviors. A major criterion of the pain treatment program is that professional intervention, whether by medication or by attention and responsiveness on the part of the therapist, must never be contingent on the experience of pain. Obviously, this approach may conflict with other forms of intervention being used with the patient, and collaboration with other health care professionals is mandatory.

For patients referred for behavioral intervention, pain behaviors must be pinpointed and the methods of communicating pain to significant others clarified. A number of steps are involved. Baseline measures of pain behaviors, usually made up of self-reports, are obtained. These include scaling the extent of pain experienced throughout a twenty-four-hour period. Frontalis tension readings are taken for an initial ten-minute period. Auditory and visual feedback are employed as the patient imagines anxiety-provoking and -alleviating scenes. Evaluation of the time sequence of activities relating to the onset of pain, its maintenance, and its termination is necessary. Distinguishing sporadic from steady pain and identifying the environmental consequences of the pain are essential aspects of the behavioral assessment procedure. The health care professional must take special care to consider nighttime behaviors; for example, does a person who cannot sleep because of pain take medication or receive extra attention from his spouse, i.e., does he receive direct positive reinforcement? Specification of the verbal and nonverbal communication of pain enables one to note the antecedent and consequent events of pain behavior. The treater must carefully analyze how the patient is reinforced for pain behavior. He must assess pain activators — situations and events that elicit pain behaviors — and pain diminishers — those that decrease pain — so that hypotheses about the elimination of pain behaviors and the potential restoration of well behaviors may be formulated. If tension or anxiety is thought to be a reinforcement for pain, such treatments as biofeedback and relaxation should be considered. Asking the patient and spouse to describe a "typical day" before and after the onset of pain provides information about work and social and leisure activity and helps to determine whether operant or respondent factors of pain are present. Additional personality data (Fordyce, 1976) can be obtained from activity logs made up before the behavioral analysis. It is important to tell the patient that treatment does not routinely or easily eliminate the pain altogether but that a multi-focus treatment package will help the patient work on problems relating to the pain.

Under some circumstances an operant pain treatment approach is contraindicated: (1) If the appropriate positive reinforcements are not forthcoming or the spouse is resistant to participating in treatment, the environmental contingencies will remain unaltered. Thus, there can be no change in reinforcement. (2) Patients who continue to use pain medication or who are receiving substantial compensation benefits for pain probably have significant psychological difficulty and have a history of previous involvement in behavioral approaches. (See Fordyce [1976] for a detailed review of what patients are appropriate for an operant-conditioning program and Devine and

Merskey [1965] for an assessment of the personalities of pain patients who request intervention.)

The generalizability of well behaviors learned in the laboratory or treatment setting is a crucial issue in pain intervention. The ability to integrate newly learned responses into one's daily routine is one basis for evaluating the outcome of the intervention. The health care professional can encourage the pain patient to take responsibility for his own treatment from the outset by asking him to identify and arrange his reinforcements. Modification of the patient's natural environment to increase the number of reinforcements that serve to maintain the newly learned well behaviors is essential. Ways of accomplishing this – in particular, including the spouse or significant other in the intervention – have already been discussed. The behaviors of special concern to pain patients are medication use and daily activity. To ensure that the patient will continue to be medication-free, he should actively avoid situations that are associated with pain and are apt to reinforce drug use. The implicit assumption is that medication-taking behavior is reinforced continually in the patient's environment. Follow-up booster sessions with the therapist are helpful in strengthening more constructive behavior. The patient should continue the activity and exercise program started during intervention so that reinforcement occurs through mastering the exercise quotas. Charting daily exercise is recommended to give ongoing feedback on performance and elicit social reinforcement. The type of exercise was narrowly defined at the onset of treatment; a gradual broadening can now be encouraged to include enjoyable vocational and leisure activities. It is important for both the clinician and patient to acknowledge that flare-ups of pain may occur long after the end of intervention. Active treatment may be appropriate at this time, but it is likely to be short-lived and to consist of additional training for the spouse or significant other and the reinstitution of exercise quotas. Careful review of the situation may reveal a source of operant pain. The gain already made in treatment should then be reestablished and strengthened.

As members of the health care team, physicians and nurses come into contact with pain patients at a particularly important time. In addition, by virtue of their professional status, they are likely to have special problems relating to the management of these patients. Implicit in the physician-patient relationship is the patient's hope for a solution to the pain and for a quick recovery. The patient both expects and demands rapid resolution. He continues to demand action from his physician if initial efforts to reduce the pain are not successful. The temptation to yield to the patient and prescribe pain medication is real, yet the use of such medications can lead to habituation, addiction, and the reinforcement of pain behavior. With self-restraint, the physician can treat the patient in a more appropriate fashion, using the behavioral principles outlined in this section.

The patient's tendency to call the physician when he experiences intolerable pain and the physician's responsiveness tend merely to strengthen pain behavior. The physician's attention has become pain-contingent. It is essential that the physician be knowledgeable about the conditions that produce operant pain, in particular to the risks involved in giving "attention as needed."

Nurses are primarily responsible for the ongoing care and management of in-patients. Those with chronic pain syndromes need "deconditioning" of the maladaptive pain behaviors. Behaviors apparently incompatible with pain, such as goal-directed activity and social interaction, should be praised openly, and pain behaviors should be ignored by the nursing staff at all times. Group therapy led by nurses is a helpful adjunct to the operant program described by Fordyce because it offers the opportunity for patients to air their feelings. Patients start to sense that they are not alone and to understand that their pain behavior does in fact elicit some payoff. They can gradually realize that the pain behaviors are a means of control. They are encouraged to perceive themselves as active collaborators rather than passive recipients in the treatment process.

In summary, behavioral intervention is appropriate for pain disorders, especially those of a chronic nature. Behavioral strategies—modification of pain behaviors and decrease in muscle-tension levels—teach the patient to function better in the environment in spite of the perception of mild to severe pain. However, these strategies also lead to a significant reduction in pain for many individuals. These methods should be considered by the health care professional when surgical or medical treatment is unwarranted and when the pain experience is part of a chronic pain syndrome in which pain is unresponsive to other intervention and persists over a long period.

There are several unresolved problems concerning the use of biofeedback with pain patients. We do not understand the precise physiological changes that occur as biofeedback training gradually decreases pain. Are the physiological changes evident during intervention secondary (i.e., are they a function of symptom change?) or primary (i.e., do they cause the symptom change?)? The relationship between the response that the patient learns to control and the physiological mechanisms responsible for the pain experience has not been delineated. As there is so little follow-up data from both biofeedback and operant programs, it is not clear whether patients can actually learn to control target behaviors. If so, how long is the control effective? And, finally, the role of placebo must be considered. Although the biofeedback technician characteristically remains neutral and objective, the attention paid to the patient may nevertheless be a powerful variable. It is likely that biofeedback treatment needs to be assessed in the context of changes in the patient's attitude toward problems, coping styles, development of life-management skills, and motivation for treatment that requires the patient to be active.

Pain is a complex phenomenon. It depends on sensory input and numerous psychological factors. Clarifying these factors would be a step further in developing a practical approach to modifying pain behavior using personality variables. The research literature does not adequately consider how to prepare people for pain, although a person's psychological status would appear to provide an important basis for determining the best approach. More work needs to be done on the assessment of subjective pain and pain behaviors. Systematic, controlled research on the effectiveness of specific behavioral treatment strategies—for example, desensitization, stress innoculation, relaxation, and biofeedback—would be valuable. Another important question is the precise relationship between personality variables and the psychological aspects of pain, including threshold, subjective experience, and pain behavior.

Up to this point, behavioral intervention has been the primary focus. In the next chapter, the issue of compliance with the recommended intervention will be discussed. Two primary models of compliance will be presented, one emphasizing the importance of altering the patient's expectations and cognitions, and the other stressing the relevance of antecedent and consequent events in the application of stimulus control to compliance behavior. Suggestions for the enhancement of compliance behavior will be presented.

BIBLIOGRAPHY

Abraham, J. L., and Allen, G. J. Comparative effectiveness of situational programming, financial payoffs, and group pressure in weight reduction. *Behavior Therapy,* 1974, 5:391–400.

Adams, E., Feuerstein, M., and Fowler, J. L. Migraine headache: Review of parameters, etiology, and intervention. *Psychological Bulletin,* 1980, 87: 217–237.

Armstrong, J. D. The search for the alcoholic personality. *Annals of the American Academy of Political and Social Science,* 1959, 315:40–42.

Azrin, N. H., Holz, W., and Goldiamond, I. Response bias in questionnaire reports. *Journal of Consulting Psychology,* 1961, 25:324–326.

Bakal, D. A. Headache: A biosocial perspective. Psychological Bulletin, 1975, 78:369–382.

Bakal, D. A., and Kaganev, J. A. Muscle contraction and migraine headache: Psychophysiological comparison. *Headache,* 1977, 7:208–217.

Bandura, A. *Principles of behavior modification.* New York: Holt, Rinehart and Winston, 1969.

———. Self-efficacy: Towards a unifying theory of behavioral change. *Psychological Review,* 1977, 84:191–215.

Beaty, E. T., and Haynes, S. N. Behavioral intervention with muscle contraction headache: A review. *Psychosomatic Medicine,* 1979, 41(2):169–175.

Beck, A. T. *Cognitive therapy and the emotional disorders.* New York: International Universities Press, 1976.

Bellack, A. S., Rozensky, R., and Schwartz, J. A comparison of 2 forms of self-monitoring in a behavioral weight reduction program. *Behavior Therapy,* 1974, 5:523–530.

Bellur, A. S. *Fat or thin: A natural history of obesity.* New York: Farrar, Straus and Giroux, 1977.

Benson, H. *The Relaxation Response.* New York: Morrow, 1975.

Benson, H., Beary, J. B., and Carol, M. The relaxation response. *Psychiatry,* 1974, 37:37–40.

Benson, H., Shapiro, D., and Tursky, B. Decreased systolic blood pressure through operant conditioning techniques in patients with essential hypertension. *Science,* 1971, 173:740–742.

Berg, R. L. The high cost of self-deception. *Preventive Medicine,* 1976, 5:483–495.

Bernard, J. L. Rapid treatment of gross obesity by operant techniques. *Psychological Reports,* 1968, 23:663–666.

Bishop, H. F. A comparison of selected biofeedback techniques in treating chronic onset insomniacs. Unpublished Ph.D. dissertation, Nova University, 1975.

Blanchard, E. B., and Young, L. D. Self-control of cardiac functioning: A promise as yet unfulfilled. *Psychological Bulletin,* 1973, 79:145-163.

_____.Clinical applications of biofeedback training . A review of evidence. *Archives of General Psychiatry,* 1974, 30:573-584.

Bootzin, R. Stimulus control of insomnia. Paper presented at a symposium on the treatment of sleep disorders at the annual meeting of the American Psychological Association, Montreal, 1973.

Bootzin, R. R. Stimulus control treatment for insomnia. Paper presented at the 80th annual convention of the American Psychological Association, Honolulu, Hawaii, 1972.

Borkovec, T. D. Pseudo (experimental) insomnia and idiopathic (objective) insomnia: Theoretical and therapeutic issues. *Advances in Behavior Research,* 1979, 2:27.

Borkovec, T. D., and Fowles, D. C. A controlled investigation of the effects of progressive and hypnotic relaxation on insomnia. *Journal of Abnormal Psychology,* 1973, 82:153-158.

Borkovec, T. D., Steinmark, S., and Nau, J. Relaxation training and single item desensitization in the group treatment of insomnia. *Journal of Behavior Therapy and Experimental Psychiatry,* 1973, 4:401-403.

Brady, J. P., Luborsky, L., and Kron, R. E. Blood pressure reduction in patients with essential hypertension through metronome-conditioned relaxation: A preliminary report. *Behavior Therapy,* 1974, 5:203-209.

Budzynski, T. H. Biofeedback in the treatment of muscle-contraction headaches. *Biofeedback and Self-Regulation,* 1978, 3(4):301-310.

Budzynski, T. H., and Stoyva, J. M. Biofeedback techniques in behavior therapy. In D. Shapiro, T. K. Barber, L. V. DiCara, J. Kamiya, N. Miller, J. Stoyva (Eds.), *Biofeedback and self-control,* 1972, (Chicago: Aldine, 1973), pp. 59-74.

Budzynski, T. H., Stoyva, J., and Adler, C. Feedback-induced relaxation: Application to tension headaches. *Journal of Behavior Therapy and Experimental Psychiatry,* 1970, 1:205-211.

Budzynski, T. H., Stoyva, J. M., and Mullaney, D. J. EMG biofeedback and tension headache: A controlled outcome study. *Psychosomatic Medicine,* 1973, 35:484-496.

Byassee, J., Farr, S., and Meyer, R. Progressive relaxation and autogenic training in the treatment of essential hypertension. Unpublished manuscript, 1976.

Cautela, J. R. Treatment of compulsive behavior by covert sensitization. *Psychological Records,* 1968, 16:33-41.

Chesney, M. A., and Shelton, J. L. A comparison of muscle relaxation and EMG feedback treatment for muscle-contraction headaches. *Journal of Behavior Therapy and Experimental Psychiatry,* 1976, 7:221-225.

Cox, D., Freundlich, A., and Meyer, R. Differential effectiveness of EMG feedback, relaxation instructions, and medication placebo with tension headaches. *Journal of Consulting and Clinical Psychology,* 1975, 43:892–898.

Cuddy, G. R., Addington, H. J., and Perkins, D. Individualized behavior therapy for alcoholics. A 3rd year of independent double-blind follow-up. Unpublished manuscript, 1978.

Cushman, O., Gray, M. G., and Moore, M. Notes on the personality of patients with migraine. *Journal of Nervous and Mental Disease,* 1943, 97:50–62.

D'Alessio, D. J. *Wolff's headache and other head pain.* New York: Oxford University Press, 1972.

Deabler, H. L., Fidel, E., and Dillenkoffer, R. L. The use of relaxation and hypnosis in lowering high blood pressure. *American Journal of Clinical Experimental Hypnosis,* 1973, 16:75–83.

Devine, R., and Merskey, H. The description of pain in psychiatric and general medical patients. *Psychosomatic Research,* 1965, 9:311.

Diamond, S., and Baltes, B. J. The diagnosis and treatment of headaches. *Chicago Medical School Quarterly,* 1973, 32(1–4).

Elder, S. T., and Eustis, N. K. Instruments of blood pressure conditioning in out-patient hypertensives. *Behavior Research and Therapy,* 1975, 13:185–188.

Ellis, A. *Reason and emotion in psychotherapy.* New York: Lyle Stuart, 1962.

Epstein, L. H., and Abel, G. G. An analysis of biofeedback training effects for tension headache patients. *Behavior Therapy,* 1977, 8:37–47.

Evans, D., and Bond, I. Reciprocal inhibition. Therapy and classical conditioning in the treatment of insomnia. *Behavior Research and Therapy,* 1969, 7:315–316.

Fahrion, S. L. Autogenic biofeedback treatment for migraine. *Mayo Clinical Proceedings,* 1977, 52:776–784.

Ferster, C. B., Nurnberger, J. I., and Levitt, E. B. The control of eating. *Journal of Mathetics,* 1962, 2:87–109.

Fordyce, W. E. *Behavioral methods for chronic pain and illness.* St. Louis: Mosby, 1976.

Fordyce, W. E., Brena, S., deLateur, B., Holcombe, S., and Loeser, J. Relationship of patient semantic pain descriptors to physician diagnostic judgments, activity, level measures, and MMPI. *Pain,* 1978, 5:293–303.

Fordyce, W. E., Fowler, R. S., deLateur, B. An application of behavior modification technique to a problem of chronic pain. *Behavior Research and Therapy,* 1968, 6:105–107.

Fordyce, W., Fowler, R., Lehman, J., and deLateur, B. Some implications of learning in problems of chronic pain. *Journal of Chronic Disability,* 1968, 21:179–190.

Fordyce, W. E., Fowler, R. S., Lehman, J. F., deLateur, B. J., Sand, P. I., and Trieschmann, R. B. Operant conditioning in the treatment of chronic pain. *Archives of Physical Medicine and Rehabilitation,* 1973, 54: 399–408.

Foreyt, J. P., and Hagen, R. L. Covert sensitization: Conditioning or suggestion? *Journal of Abnormal Psychology,* 1973, 82:17–23.

Frankel, B. L., Patel, D. J., Horwitz, D., Fredenwald, W. T., and Gaerdner, K. R. Treatment of hypertension with biofeedback and relaxation techniques. *Psychosomatic Medicine,* 1978, 40:276–293.

Friar, L. R. Operant training with biofeedback of pulse amplitude decreases in normal and migraine subjects. Ph.D. dissertation, University of California, 1974. (Dissertation Abstracts International, 1974, 35:1046B–1048B [University Microfilms, 74-18, 700]).

Friedman, A. P. Reflection on the problem of headache. *Journal of the American Medical Association,* 1964, 190:121–123.

Fromm-Reichmann, F. Contributions to the psychogenesis of migraine. *Psychoanalytic Review,* 1937, 24.

Frumkin, K., Nathan, R. J., Prout, M. J., and Cohen, M. C. Nonpharmocologic control of essential hypertension in man: A critical review of the experimental literature. *Psychosomatic Medicine,* 1978, 40:4.

Geer, J. M., and Katkin, E. S. Treatment of insomnia using a variant of systematic desensitization: A case report. *Journal of Abnormal Psychology,* 1966, 71:161–164.

Gormally, J., Buese-Moscati, E., Clyman, R., and Forbes, R. R. Research design issues for the behavioral treatment of obesity. Abstracted in the Journal Supplement of Abstract Service (of the American Psychological Association) catalog of selected documents in *Psychology,* 1977, 7(2):34.

Green, E. G., Green, A. M., and Walters, E. D. Biofeedback for mind-body self regulation: Healing and creativity. Unpublished manuscript, available from the Research Department, Menninger Foundation, Topeka, Kansas, 1971.

Green, G., Green, A., and Walters, D. Voluntary control of internal states: Psychological and physiological. *Journal of Transpersonal Psychology,* 1970, 1:1–26.

Grenfell, R. F., Briggs, A. M., and Holland, W. C. Antihypertensive drugs: A controlled evaluation. *Journal of the Mississippi State Medical Association,* 1962, 3:93–98.

Grinker, R. Behavioral and metabolic consequences of weight reduction. *Journal of the American Dietetic Association,* 1973, 62:30–34.

Hagen, R., Foreyt, J., and Durham, C. The drop-out problem. *Behavior Therapy,* 1976, 7:463–471.

Harmatz, M. G., and Lepuc, P. Behavior modification of overeating in a psychiatric hospital. *Journal of Consulting and Clinical Psychology,* 1968, 32:583–587.

Harris, M. B. Self-directed program for weight control: A pilot study. *Journal of Abnormal Psychology,* 1969, 74:263–270.

Hauri, P. What is good sleep? In E. Hartmann (Ed.), *Sleep and dreaming* (Boston: Little, Brown, and Company, 1970), pp. 70–76.

Haynes, S., Griffin, P., Mooney, D., and Parise, M. Electromyographic feedback and relaxation instructions in the treatment of muscle-contraction headaches. *Behavior Therapy,* 1975, 6:672–678.

Henry, J. P. Relaxation methods and the control of blood pressure. *Psychosomatic Medicine,* 1978, 40:4.

Jacobson, A. *Progressive relaxation.* Chicago: University of Chicago Press, 1938.

Jeffrey, D. B. Additional methodological considerations in the behavioral treatment of obesity: A reply to the Hall and Hall review of obesity. *Behavior Therapy,* 1975, 6:96–97.

Jessor, R., and Jessor, S. L. Adolescent development and the onset of drinking: A longitudinal study. *Journal of Studies on Alcoholism,* 1975, 36:27–51.

Kalb, D. A., Winter, S. K., and Berlew, D. A. Self-directed change: 25 studies. *Journal of Applied Behavioral Science,* 1968, 4:453–476.

Kales, A., and Berger, R. J. Psychopathology of sleep. In G. G. Castello (Ed.), *Symptoms of Psychopathology* (New York: John Wiley, 1970), pp. 103–122.

Kales, A., and Kales, J. Recent advances in the diagnosis and treatment of sleep disorders. In G. Usin (Ed.), *Sleep research and clinical practice* (New York: Brunner/Mazel, 1973), pp. 61–80.

Karacan, M., and Williams, R. L. Insomnia: Old wine in a new bottle. *Psychiatric Quarterly,* 1971, 45:274–278.

Keefe, F. J. Conditioning changes in differential skin temperature. *Perceptual and Motor Skills,* 1975, 46:283–288.

Keys, A. and Grande, F. Body weight, body composition, and calorie status. In A. S. Goodhart and M. E. Shils (Eds.), *Modern nutrition in health and disease,* 5th ed. (Philadelphia: Lea and Febiger, 1973), pp. 106–141.

Kingsley, R. G., and Wilson, G. T. Behavior therapy for obesity: A comparative investigation of long-term efficacy. *Journal of Consulting and Clinical Psychology,* 1978, 45:288.

Kleinman, K. H., Goldman, H., Snow, M. Y., and Kozol, B. Effects of stress and motivation on the effectiveness of biofeedback training in essential hypertension. Paper presented at the 7th annual meetings of the Biofeedback Research Society, Colorado Springs, Colorado, 1976.

Klumbies, G., and Eberhart, G. Results of autogenic training in the treatment of hypertension. In J. J. Lopez Ibor (Ed.), *IV World Congress of Psychiatry, Madrid, 5–11 September 1966.* International Congress Series, No. 117, pp. 46–47. Amsterdam: Excerpta Medica Foundation, 1966.

Knopf, O. Preliminary report on personality studies in 30 migraine patients. *Journal of Nervous and Mental Disease,* 1935, 82:270–285.

Kolotkin, R. L. Assertion training, spouse involvement, and individual differences in a cognitive-behavioral treatment of obesity. Unpublished manuscript, University of Minnesota, 1978.

Kondo, C., and Canter, C. True and false electromyographic feedback; Effect on muscle-tension headache. *Journal of Abnormal Psychology*, 1977, 86:93–95.

Krist, D. A., and Engel, B. R. Learned control of blood pressure in patients with high blood pressure. *Circulation*, 1975, 51:370–378.

Lazarus, A. Toward the understanding and effective treatment of alcoholism. *South African Medical Journal*, 1965, 39:736–741.

_____. *Clinical behavior therapy.* New York: Brunner/Mazel, 1977.

Lazarus, A. A. Psychiatric problems precipitated by transcendental meditation. *Psychological Reports*, 1976, 39:601–602.

Leavitt, F., and Garron, D. C. Psychological disturbance and pain report differences in both organic and non-organic low back pain patients. *Pain*, 1979, 7:187–195.

Leon, G. R., and Roth, L. Obesity, psychological causes, correlations, and speculations. *Psychological Bulletin*, 1977, 84:117–139.

Lipinski, D., and Nelson, R. Problems in the use of naturalistic observation as a means of behavioral assessment. *Behavior Therapy*, 1974, 5: 341–351.

Lynn, R., and Eysenck, H. J. Tolerance for pain, extroversion, and neuroticism. *Perceptual and Motor Skills*, 1961, 12:161.

McReynolds, W. T., Lutz, R. N., Paulsen, B. K., and Kohrs, M. B. Weight loss resulting from two behavior modification procedures with nutritionists as therapists. *Behavior Therapy*, 1976, 7:283–291.

Mahoney, M. J. The behavioral treatment of obesity: A reconnaissance. *Biofeedback and Self-Regulation*, 1976, 1:127–133.

_____. Self-reward and self-monitoring techniques for weight control. *Behavior Therapy*, 1974, 5:48–57.

Mahoney, M. J., and Arnkoff, D. B. Cognitive and self-control therapies. In S. L. Garfield and A. G. Bergin (Eds.), *Handbook of psychotherapy and behavior change*, 2d ed. (New York: Wiley, 1978), pp. 661–689.

Mahoney, M. J., and Mahoney, K. Treatment of obesity: A clinical exploration. In B. J. Williams, S. Martin, and J. Foreyt (Eds.), *Obesity: Behavioral approaches to dietary management* (New York: Brunner/Mazel, 1976), pp. 30–34.

Mahoney, M. J., and Thoreson, C. E. (Eds.). *Self-control: Power to the person.* Monterey, California: Brooks/Cole, 1974.

Mann, R. A. The behavior-therapeutic use of contingency contracting to control an adult behavior problem: Weight control. *Journal of Applied Behavior Analysis*, 1972, 5:99–109.

Manno, B., and Marston, A. R. Weight reduction as a function of negative covert reinforcement (sensitization) versus positive covert reinforcement.

Behavioral Research and Therapy, 1972, 10:201–207.

Meichenbaum, D., and Turk, D. The cognitive-behavioral management of anxiety, anger, and pain. In P. Davidson (Ed.), *The behavioral management of anxiety, depression and pain* (New York: Brunner/Mazel, 1976), pp. 206–250.

Melzack, R., and Chapman, C. Psychological aspects of pain. *Postgraduate Medicine*, 1973, 53:69–75.

Merskey, H. Psychological aspects of pain. *Postgraduate Medical Journal*, 1968, 44:297–306.

Miall, W. E. Heredity and hypertension. *Practitioner*, 1971, 207:20–27.

Miller, N. Learning of visceral and glandular responses. *Science*, 1969, 163: 434.

Miller, R., and Caddy, G. Abstinence and controlled drinking in the treatment of problem drinking. *Journal of Studies of Alcohol*, 1977, 38: 986–1003.

Mitchell, K. R., and White, R. G. Self-management of tension headaches: A case study. *Journal of Behavior Therapy and Experimental Psychiatry*, 1976, 7:387–389.

Monroe, L. J. Psychological and physiological differences between good and poor sleepers. *Journal of Abnormal Psychology*, 1967, 74:255.

Nathan, P. E., and Goldman, M. S. Problem drinking and alcoholism. In G. Pomerleau and J. Brady (Eds.), *Behavioral medicine: Theory and practice* (Baltimore: Williams and Wilkins, 1979), pp. 255–277.

Nathan, P. E., and Lansky, D. Management of the chronic alcholic: A behavioral viewpoint. In J. P. Brady and H.K.H. Brodie (Eds.), *Controversy in psychiatry* (Philadelphia: W. B. Saunders, 1978), pp. 65–90.

Nessman, D. G., Carnahan, J. E., and Nugent, C. A. Increasing compliance: patient-operated hypertension groups. *Archives of Internal Medicine*, 1980, 140:1427–1430.

Nicassio, P., and Bootzin, R. A comparison of progressive relaxation and autogenic training versus treatments for insomnia. *Journal of Abnormal Psychology*, 1974, 83:253–260.

Oswald, I. Drugs and sleep. *Pharmacology Review*, 1968, 20:272–303.

Patel, C., and North, W.R.S. Randomized controlled trial of yoga and biofeedback in the management of hypertension. *Lancet*, 1975, 2:93–95.

Peper, E. Frontiers of clinical biofeedback. In L. Birk (Ed.), *Seminars in psychiatry*, 5 vols. (New York: Grune and Stratton, 1973), 5:350–352.

Philips, C. The modification of tension headache pain using EMG feedback. *Behavior Research Therapy*, 1977, 15:119–129.

Pilowsky, I. The response to treatment in hypochondriacal disorders. *Australian and New Zealand Journal of Psychiatry*, 1968, 12:88–94.

Pomerleau, O. F., and Brady, J. P. (Eds.). *Behavioral medicine: Theory and practice*. Baltimore: Williams and Wilkins, 1979.

Pomerleau, O. F., Pertschuk, M., Adkins, D., and Brady, J. P. A comparison of behavioral and traditional treatment for middle income problem drinkers. *Journal of Behavioral Medicine,* 1978, 1:187–200.

Poser, E. G., Fenton, G. W., and Scotton, L. The classical conditioning of sleep and wakefulness. *Behavior Research and Therapy,* 1965, 3:259–264.

Rachman, S. J., and Philips, C. *Psychology and behavioral medicine.* New York: Cambridge University Press, 1980.

Raskin, M., Johnson, G., and Rondertvedt, J. W. Chronic anxiety treated by feedback in direct muscle relaxation: A pilot study. *Archives of General Psychiatry,* 1973, 28:263–266.

Ribordy, S. C., and Denney, D. R. The behavioral treatment of insomnia: An alternative to drug therapy. *Behavioral Research and Therapy,* 1977, 15:39–50.

Romanczyk, R. G. Self-monitoring in the treatment of obesity: Parameters of reactivity. *Behavior Therapy,* 1974, 5:531–540.

Sainsbury, P., and Gibson, J. G. Symptoms of anxiety and tension and the accompanying physiological changes in the muscular system. *Journal of Neurology, Neurosurgery, and Psychiatry,* 1954, 17:216–224.

Sargent, J., Walters, C., and Green, E. Psychosomatic self-regulation of migraine headache. In L. Birk (Ed.), *Seminars in psychiatry,* 5 vols. (New York: Grune and Stratton, 1973), 5:415–428.

Sargent, J. D., Green, E. E., and Walters, E. D. Preliminary report on the use of autogenic feedback training in the treatment of migraine and tension headaches. *Psychosomatic Medicine,* 1973, 35:129–135.

Schachter, S. *Emotion, obesity, and crime.* New York: Academic Press, 1971.

Schachter, S., and Rodin, J. *Obese humans and rats.* Potomac, Maryland: Erlbaum, 1974.

Schmidt, W., and Popham, R. C. Heavy alcohol consumption and physical health problems: A review of the epidemiological evidence. *Drug and Alcohol Dependence,* 1975, 27–50.

Schultz, J. M., and Luthe, W. *Autogenic therapy, vol. I. Autogenic method.* New York: Grune and Stratton, 1969.

Schwartz, G. E., and Shapiro, D. Biofeedback and essential hypertension: Current findings and theoretical concerns. In L. Birk (Ed.), *Seminars in psychiatry,* 5 vols. (New York: Grune and Stratton, 1973), 5:493–503.

Seligman, M. *Helplessness.* San Francisco: W. H. Freeman, 1975.

Shapiro, A. P., Redmond, D. P., and McDonald, R. H. Relationship of perception, cognition, and operant conditioning in essential hypertension. *Progress in Brain Research,* 1975, 42:299–312.

Shapiro, A. P., Schwartz, G. E., and Ferguson, D.C.E. Behavioral methods in the treatment of hypertension. *Northeastern Medicine,* 1977, 86:626–636.

Shapiro, B., Benson, H., Tursky, B., and Schwartz, G. E. Decreased systolic blood pressure through operant conditioning techniques in patients with essential hypertension. *Science*, 1971, 173:740–742.

Shapiro, D., Schwartz, G. E., and Benson, H. Biofeedback: A behavioral approach to cardiovascular self-control. In R. S. Elliot (Ed.), *Contemporary problems in cardiology, vol. 1. Stress and the heart* (Mount Kisco, New York: Futura Publishing Company, 1974), pp. 241–259.

Shapiro, D., Tursky, B., and Schwartz, G. E. Control of blood pressure in man by operant conditioning. *Circulation Research*, 1970, 27:27–32.

Sobell, M. B., and Sobell, L. C. Alcoholics treated by individualized behavior therapy: 1 year treatment outcome. *Behavioral Research and Theory*, 1973, 11:599–618.

Southerland, E. H., Schroeder, H. G., and Tordella, C. L. Personality traits and the alcoholic. *Quarterly Journal Studies of Alcoholism*, 1950, 11:547–561.

Spear, F. Pain in psychiatric patients. *Journal of Psychosomatic Research*, 1967, 11:187–193.

Steger, J., and Harper, R. EMG biofeedback versus in vivo self-monitored relaxation in the treatment of tension headaches. Paper presented at the annual meeting of the Western Psychological Association, Seattle, April 1977.

Steinmark, S. W., and Borkovec, T. D. In T. D. Borkovec and D. A. Bernstein (Eds.), *Progressive relaxation training* (Chicago: Research Press, 1973).

Sternbach, R., Wolf, S., Murphy, R., and Wolfe, S. Aspects of low back pain. *Postgraduate Medicine*, 1973, 53:226–229.

Sternbach, R. A. *Pain: A psychophysiological analysis.* New York: Academic Press, 1968.

_____. *Pain patients: Traits and treatment.* New York: Academic Press, 1974a.

_____. Varieties of pain games. In J. J. Bonica (Ed.), *Advances in neurology, vol. 4, Pain* (New York: Raven Press, 1974b).

Sternbach, R. A., and Fordyce, W. Psychogenic pain. In J. J. Bonica (Ed.), *The management of pain*, 2d ed. (Philadelphia: Lea and Febiger, 1975), pp. 71–80.

Sternbach, R. A., and Tursky, B. Ethnic differences among housewives in psychophysiological and skin potential responses to electric shock. *Psychophysiology*, 1965, 1:241–246.

Stone, R. A., and DeLeo, J. Psychotherapeutic control of hypertension. *New England Medical Journal*, 1976, 294:80–84.

Stoyva, J., and Budzynski, J. Cultivated low-arousal—an anti-stress response. In L. V. DiCara (Ed.), *Limbic and autonomic nervous system research* (New York: Plenum, 1974).

Stroebel, C. F., and Glueck, B. C. Biofeedback treatment in medicine and psychiatry: An ultimate placebo? In L. Birk (Ed.), *Seminars in psychiatry, 5* vols. (New York: Grune and Stratton, 1973), 5:379–393.

Stuart, R. B. Behavioral control of overeating. *Behavior Research and Therapy,* 1967, 5:357–365.

_____. A three dimensional program for the treatment of obesity. *Behavior Research and Therapy,* 1971, 9:177–186.

Stuart, R. B., and Davis, B. *Slim chance in a fat world: Behavioral control of obesity.* Champaign, Illinois: Research Press, 1972.

Stunkard, A. New therapies for the eating disorders: Behavior modification of obesity and anorexia nervosa. *Archives of General Psychiatry,* 1972, 26:391–398.

Stunkard, A. J., Levine, H., and Fox, S. The management of obesity: Patient self-help and medical treatment. *Archives of Internal Medicine,* 1970, 125:1067–1072.

Stunkard, A. J., and McLaren-Hume, M. The results of treatment for obesity: A review of the literature and report of a series. *Archives of Internal Medicine,* 1959, 103:79–85.

Stunkard, A. J., and Mahoney, M. J. Behavioral treatment of eating disorders. In H. Leitenberg (Ed.), *Handbook of behavior modification* (New York: Appleton-Century-Crofts, 1976), pp. 45–76.

Stunkard, A. J., and Rush, J. Dieting and depression reexamined: A critical review of reports of untoward responses during weight reduction for obesity. *Annals of Internal Medicine,* 1974, 81:526–533.

Suczek, R. F. Psychological aspects of weight reduction. In E. S. Eppfight, P. Swanson, and G. A. Inversson (Eds.), *Weight Control: A collection of papers presented at the Weight Control Colloquium* (Ames: Iowa State University Press, 1955).

Syme, L. Personality studies of the alcoholic. *Quarterly Journal Studies of Alcohol,* 1957, 18:288–301.

Tarter-Benidio, L. The role of relaxation in biofeedback training: A critical review of the literature. *Psychological Bulletin,* 1978, 83:727–755.

Taub, E., and Emurian, C. S. Operant control of skin temperature. Paper presented at the meeting of the Biofeedback Research Society, St. Louis, 1971.

Thompson, R. F., and Patterson, M. M. (Eds.). *Bioelectric recording techniques, Vol. 1, Part C, Receptor and effector processes.* New York: Academic Press, 1974.

Thoreson, C. E., and Mahoney, M. J. *Behavioral self-control.* New York: Holt, Rinehart and Winston, 1974.

Turin, A., and Johnson, W. G. Biofeedback therapy for migraine headaches. *Archives of General Psychiatry,* 1976, 38:517–519.

Turk, D. Cognitive-behavioral techniques in the management of pain. In J. Foreyt and D. Rathjen (Eds.), *Cognitive behavior therapy: Research and implications* (New York:Plenum, 1978), pp. 61-72.

Tursky, B., Shapiro, O., and Schwartz, G. E. Automated constant self-pressure system to measure average systolic and diastolic blood pressure in man. *IEEE Transportation Biomedical Engineering,* 1972, 19:271–276.

Ullmann, L. P., and Krasner, L. (Eds.). *Case studies in behavior modification.* New York: Holt, Rinehart and Winston, 1965.

Van Boxtel, A., and Vander Ven, J. R. Differential EMG activity in subjects with muscle-contraction headaches related to mental effort. *Headache,* 1978, 17:233–237.

Vaughn, R., Pall, M. L., and Haynes, S. N. Frontalis EMG response to stress in subjects with frequent muscle-contraction headaches. *Headache,* 1977, 16:313–317.

Weisenberg, M. Pain and pain control. *Psychological Bulletin,* 1977, 84:1008–1044.

Weiss, A. R. A behavioral approach to the treatment of adolescent obesity. *Behavior Therapy,* 1977, 8:720–726.

Wickramasekera, I. The application of verbal instructions and EMG feedback training to the management of tension-headache – preliminary investigations. *Headache,* 1973, 13:74–76.

_____. Instruction and EMG biofeedback with systematic desensitization: A case report. *Behavior Therapy,* 1972, 3:460–465.

Williams, R. B., and Gentry, W. D. *Behavioral approaches to medical treatment.* Cambridge, Massachusetts: Ballinger, 1977.

Wilson, G. T. Alcoholism and aversion therapy: Issues, ethics, and evidence. In G. A. Marlatt and P. E. Nathan (Eds.), *Behavioral assessment and treatment of alcoholism* (New Brunswick, New Jersey: Rutgers Center of Alcohol Studies, 1978a).

_____. Behavioral treatment of obesity: Maintenance, strategies, and long-term efficacy. Unpublished manuscript, 1978b.

Wollersheim, J. P. Effectiveness of group therapy based on learning principles in the treatment of overweight women. *Journal of Abnormal Psychology,* 1970, 76:462–474.

Wolpe, J. *Headache and other head pain.* New York: Oxford University Press, 1972.

Wolpe, J., and Lang, P. J. A fear survey schedule for use in behavior therapy. *Behavior Research and Therapy,* 1964, 2:27–30.

Woodforde, J., and Merskey, H. Personality traits of patients with chronic pain. *Journal of Psychosomatic Research,* 1972, 16:167.

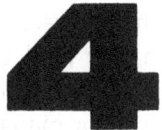

COMPLIANCE BEHAVIOR

INTRODUCTION

Compliance behavior can be defined as "cooperation with the recommendations of health care personnel" (Counte and Christman, 1981:63) or "the consistency of patient behavior with a program of treatment as prescribed by a medical authority" (Salloway, Pletcher, and Collins, 1978:103). Fabrega (1975:972) described compliance in the following way:

> In a rather basic sense, medical practitioners regardless of culture have to persuade people to do such things as take medication, alter personal habits, agree to submit to dangerous proceedings, acknowledge negative personality attributes, modify their relationships with others, accept and reorient themselves to bodily constraints, return for follow-up visits, comply with and participate in formally structured exchanges, check and report on bodily functions, and so forth.

Getting a patient to cooperate with a prescribed ongoing treatment program is a sigificant problem for the clinician. The patient may refuse to adhere to therapeutic instructions by not taking the prescribed medication or by not participating in recommended activity. The long-term effect of such noncompliance is, of course, the inability to maintain whatever good result, however minimal, was initially obtained and in some cases, such as hypertension, substantial medical risk for the patient. Another book in this series, *Interpersonal Behavior and Health Care* (Counte and Christman, 1981), offers a complete discussion of compliance as an aspect of the interaction between patient and health care provider. The authors consider theoretical approaches that explain patient noncompliance, patient attitudes toward medical treatment and facilities, and the quality of the interaction between health care professionals and patients, which directly affects patient satisfaction and compliance. In this chapter I will outline behavioral strategies to maximize the potential for compliance and offer specific techniques based on these strategies for managing the noncompliant patient.

There have been many reports estimating the frequency and prevalence of noncompliance behavior (Sackett and Snow, 1979). Two warrant discussion here. Korsch and Negrete (1972) studied the mothers of children brought to the emergency room of a local hospital. Although they reported satisfaction with the E.R., most mothers were ignorant of the causes of their children's illnesses and assumed that they had been negligent in providing for their children. Forty-two percent complied with the treating physician's advice, and there seemed to be a close association between the mother's satisfaction with the consultation and compliance. There was no apparent correlation between the length of the consultation and the satisfaction of the mother or between the length of the visit and diagnostic clarity. The mothers generally described the physicians as distant, excessively caught up in medical jargon, and unsympathetic. In a second report, Ley (1977) reviewed sixty-eight studies of compliance. He found that only a little more than half the patients followed their physician's advice. The majority ignored the advice even when it was presented as crucial to their health. One of the most frequent complaints about physicians is that they do a poor job of communicating with their patients. As the trend in medicine moves away from primary care and toward specialization, the trusting relationship between patient and professional deteriorates. The number of visits to physicians has increased, but visits tend to be shorter and more symptom-oriented. The role of psychological variables in this interaction is overlooked; noncompliance may frequently be the result of the troubled clinician-patient relationship.

COMPLIANCE AND NONCOMPLIANCE

There are different forms of compliance that are not correlated with each other. Patients who say they will comply with their physicians' advice do not necessarily do so. Compliance behavior cannot be predicted from demographic and socioeconomic characteristics. Rather, compliance is associated more with features of the procedures or regimens to be followed. Noncompliance results from social variables over which the patient has little or no control. Thus, patients who are passive, used to yielding automatically to authority, and oriented to immediate gratification will be likely to resist making changes in habits—reducing the frequency of alcohol and nicotine use, for example—but will find it easier to follow recommendations for medication use. Kasl (1975) viewed noncompliance as a behavioral problem influenced by learning. The emphasis in this model is on the need to change the patient's cognition and expectations of the proposed treatment before trying to directly modify the noncompliance.

Zifferblatt (1975) viewed compliance as a behavior. As such, it is a function of antecedent events and consequent events. Antecedent events, or cues, tell a patient what needs to be done. When cues are positive, compliance behavior is very high; negative cues yield less compliance. Use of medication is an example: Medications with highly unpleasant side effects (cues) will result in inadequate compliance. If the patient feels better after initial use of medication, compliance behavior is apt to increase. If taking medication is associated with neither good nor bad outcome (i.e., the patient sees no concrete effects of the medication), a low probability of compliance is likely. Zifferblatt noted that cues must have three characteristics in order to affect compliance behavior positively—salience, compatibility with the patient's routine, and clarity.

Zifferblatt specified two steps in the enhancement of compliance behavior. The first, determining the problem, requires special attention to specific patient behavior. In particular, visual access to target behavior is necessary; for example, seeing someone taking medication is preferable to relying on his report. It is essential that the patient understand precisely which behavior constitutes compliance and which outcome signifies successful treatment. Identification of events that precede or follow the target behavior is necessary so that the prescribed treatment regimen can be adjusted as much as possible to the patient's routine; this should increase the probability of adherence. Thus, the clinician must structure his interaction with the patient and recommend specific, concrete activities. The clinician can make definite suggestions about compliance and still take the patient's needs into account. It is essential that the clinician provide confirmation to the patient about his condition as well as help him to adopt the necessary self-correcting procedures. The effects of intervention must be continually assessed so that events can be manipulated until the satisfactory outcome – full compliance – is obtained.

The second step in affecting compliance behavior consists of teaching the patient to take responsibility for the management of the problem. Self-observation, goal-setting, determination of realistic means to achieve the goal, and evaluation of outcome all allow the patient to assume a major role in determining (in collaboration with his physician) how to approach a specific medical problem. According to this view, the physician is a resource for the patient.

Tailoring treatment to the patient's regular routine is essential. Thus, the physician should arrange convenient appointment hours for the patient; the responsibility for keeping the appointment should then be the patient's. The more self-control is experienced or perceived by the patient, the better the chance of compliance. Noncompliance is frequently dismissed as a result of lack of motivation; however, noncompliance or partial compliance should never be taken lightly. The physician should suggest self-management techniques when appropriate and help the patient to identify compliance-related events and determine strategies to effect compliance. Most important, the physician should provide the patient with a more informed role in his health and health care.

The disparity between patient expectations and actual experience of the treatment process may cause noncompliance or even termination of the recommended treatment. Goldfried and Davidson (1976) stated that shaping expectations that are consistent with the anticipated outcome of treatment promotes adherence to treatment. Structuring the treatment process generally enhances compliance behavior. The procedures involved in structuring are exploring the problem, identifying it fully for the patient, explaining why the prescribed regimen is appropriate, and outlining the patient's responsibility in his treatment (Goldfried and Davidson, 1976). An essential variable to consider is the complexity of the treatment regimen. Complicated or stressful programs must be introduced gradually so that the patient can assimilate each step at his own rate. During a medical crisis, there will be little chance for the physician to attend to the issue of compliance. At such times, it may be necessary to delegate this task to other members of the health care team after the acute phase of treatment.

In summary, Zifferblatt has formulated a stimulus control, or cue technique, approach to increasing compliance behavior in health care. He viewed noncompliant behavior as the expression of beliefs and attitudes that counter those of the physician. Both Kasl and Zif-ferblatt agreed that physicians are probably not the best people to work with patients to enhance compliance because of their heavy time and patient commitments. Brief encounters with the patient in which the physician blithely states "you have to take care of yourself" do not promote automatic compliance. Encouraging the patient to participate in self-management programs and to internalize antecedent and consequent events will improve compliance.

INCREASING COMPLIANCE

Early attempts to facilitate compliance consisted of operant conditioning procedures, including reinforcement, shaping, and contingency contracting (Zifferblatt, 1975). Taking medication compliance as an example, the problem must first be defined in terms of current behavior and the related events preceding and succeeding the use of medication. Timing of the intervention and fitting it into the patient's daily routine are important in increasing the probability of compliance. If taking medication is followed by pleasing or reinforcing consequences, the probability will be increased.

Other aspects of treatment are also important. The clinician must gain the patient's trust so that the patient can openly express his thoughts and feelings without fear of criticism. Satisfactory communication and discussion enable the clinician to give feedback to the patient under nonstressful conditions. Physicians who are warm, empathic, and at ease socially are likely to obtain a high level of compliance. Further, use of specific, concrete instructions that are geared to the intellectual level of the patient and demonstration of continuing interest and genuine concern on the part of the physician will clearly lead to compliance behavior. It is essential that the clinician build in the expectation of a positive outcome. The immediate consequences of an event control behavior better than do delayed consequences.

Medication that has very unpleasant side effects is apt to cause decreased compliance regardless of the anticipated long-term outcome (Blackwell, 1973), but the physician can compensate for the negative impact by maintaining an optimistic attitude. Rates of noncompliance with prescribed medication are high. At times, poor communication by the patient with his physician is associated with noncompliance. Just as the physician may be a frequent reminder to the patient of his failure to undergo successful treatment, so too ineffective treatments by themselves lead to poor compliance. With noncompliance, consideration of three factors is essential: (1) the patient's unwillingness or inability to comply with instructions; (2) fear of social disapproval; and (3) anticipation of failure causing a decrease in motivation in the absence of prior failures. Direct training and rehearsal of compliant behaviors as part of a structured intervention may help reduce noncompliance.

To increase compliance, the patient's psychological resistance must be reduced (Brehm, 1966). The physician or other health care professional should detail the desired behavior to the patient and collaborate with the patient in working out a stepwise approach to accomplish the goal. It is important that the patient commit himself from the outset to a well-defined task; a formal contact may be useful in some cases. Gradually offering information about treatment prevents the patient from feeling overwhelmed and confused. The patient's daily activity must be disrupted as little as possible. In addition, the physician must ensure that compliance with care regimen does not interfere with another plan. Perhaps the best description of the doctor-patient relationship with respect to compliance is that the physician provides expertise within a problem-solving interaction. The physician should foster a sense of self-attribution on the part of the patient so that any improvement that occurs as a result of compliance with the prescribed regimen is perceived as a consequence of the patient's own behavior.

SUMMARY AND OVERVIEW

Compliance encompasses a complex set of behaviors that relate to the ability to adhere to a prescribed treatment plan. Characteristics of the clinician and the patient and the interaction between the two influence compliance. Both Kasl and Zifferblatt formulated models that include the contingencies yielding the highest rate of compliance. It is essential to identify the antecedents of compliance behavior that elicit adherence to the prescribed treatment plan and the behavioral consequences of following treatment (Pomerleau and Brady, 1979). Physicians who have little time to help recalcitrant patients may attempt to restructure their approach so as to enhance compliance, but the resulting tendency to work under pressure, with little time, may actually decrease compliance.

Demographic and socioeconomic variables do influence compliance behavior (see Counte and Christman, 1981). The ability to understand and recall the details of the treatment regimen and satisfaction with the treater have a strong effect as well. Compliance is clearly apt to be better when the clinician is available, understanding, and positive about treatment. Dunbar and Stunkard (1967) provided specific recommendations for improving compliance: (1) education of the patient about the treatment plan and its rationale; (2) use of self-monitoring techniques; and (3) adaptation of desired behaviors to the patient's daily activity. Treating patients at the patient's place of work provides valuable social support from colleagues and is thus likely to increase compliance.

The more complex the treatment regimen, the poorer the compliance. Thus, frequent consultation with other health care professionals is necessary. Hospitalization may be recommended, in part to permit further assessment of a problem in the structured in-patient setting and in part to institute treatment for very difficult or resistant patients. Thus, the physician needs to know about the health care within the hospital and acceptable methods of referral and collaboration. (The physician-patient relationship will be discussed in Chapter 5.) The appropriateness of psychiatric and psychological consultation as well as alternative treatment or management approaches in the medical center must be considered. Physicians must be able to identify patients who are most suitable for psychiatric and psychological consultation and must understand the nature of the referral process.

BIBLIOGRAPHY

Blackwell, B. Patient compliance. *New England Journal of Medicine,* 1973, 289:249–253.

Brehm, J. W. *A theory of psychological reactance.* New York: Academic Press, 1966.

Counte, M. A. and Christman, L. P. *Interpersonal behavior and health care.* Boulder, Colorado: Westview Press, 1981.

Caron, H. S., and Roth, H. P. Patients' cooperation with a medical regimen. *Journal of the American Medical Association,* 1968, 203:120–124.

Davidson, P. O., and Davidson, S. M. (Eds.). *Behavioral medicine: Changing health lifestyles.* New York: Brunner/Mazel, 1980.

Davis, M. S. Variation in patients' compliance with doctor's orders: Medical practice and doctor-patient interaction. *Psychiatric Medicine,* 1971, 2:31–53.

Dunbar, J., and Stunkard, A. J. Adherence to diet and drug regimen. In R.

Levey, B. Rifkind, B. Dennis, and N. Ernst (Eds.), *Nutrition, lipids, and coronary heart disease* (New York: Raven Press, 1967), pp. 102–141.

Fabrega, H. The need for ethnomedical science. *Science,* 1975, 189:969–975.

Goldfried, M. R., and Davidson, G. C. *Clinical behavior therapy.* New York: Holt, Rinehart and Winston, 1976.

Haynes, B. A critical review of the determinants of compliance. McMaster University Medical Center, Hamilton, Ontario, Canada, Workshop/Symposium: Proceedings, May 22–24, 1974.

Kasl, S. U. Issues in patient adherence to health care regimens. *Journal of Human Stress,* 1975, 1:5–17.

Korsch, B., and Negrete, M. Doctor-patient communication. *Scientific American,* 1972, 227:66–73.

Korsch, B. M., and Francis, V. Gaps in doctor-patient communication. *New England Journal of Medicine,* 1969, 280:535–540.

Ley, P. Psychological studies of doctor-patient communication. In S. Rachman (Ed.), *Contributions to medical psychology,* vol. 1 (Oxford: Pergamon Press, 1977), pp. 9–42.

Marston, M. V. Compliance with medical regimens, a review of the literature. *Nursing Research,* 1970, 19:312–323.

Pomerleau, O. F., and Brady, J. P. (Eds.). *Behavioral medicine: Theory and practice.* Baltimore: Williams and Wilkins, 1979.

Sackett, D. L., and Snow, J. L. The magnitude of compliance and noncompliance. In R. B. Haynes, D. W. Taylor, and D. L. Sackett (Eds.), *Compliance in health care* (Baltimore: Johns Hopkins University Press, 1979), p. 11.

Salloway, J. C., Pletcher, W. R., and Collins, J. J. Sociological and social psychological models of compliance with prescribed regimen: In search of synthesis. *Sociological Symposium,* 1978, 23:103.

Zifferblatt, S. M. Increasing patient compliance through the applied analysis of behavior. *Preventive Medicine,* 1975, 4:173–182.

HOSPITALIZATION: MANAGEMENT, REFERRAL, AND CONSULTATION

INTRODUCTION

Previous chapters have focused on the treatment of psychophysiological disorders (e.g., headache) and medical problems with psychological antecedents and consequences (e.g., alcoholism, obesity). Another group of patients to be considered are those who are faced with significant medical illness or who must be hospitalized. In this chapter the psychological status and needs of these patients and alternative ways of managing them will be discussed. The hospital offers many possibilities for both behavioral and more traditional intervention within its structured setting, and the health care professional needs to be familiar with the referral and consultation process. Psychology and psychiatry, despite their differences in approach, share responsibility for these procedures so that knowledge of the role of each discipline is helpful. Behavioral intervention is conducted today in hospitals, but it is most frequently integrated into the procedures of the floors on which the patients are hospitalized. It is thus difficult to control all the possible reinforcements that surround the patient. A few hospital units have been established solely for the treatment of psychophysiological disorders. The rationale, goals, procedures, and outcome for one such setting will be described in detail as a model for future behavioral intervention units.

THE PSYCHOLOGICAL IMPACT OF HOSPITALIZATION

Until recently, the psychological impact of medical illness and hospitalization was acknowledged but ignored. Now, illness and hospitalization are recognized as major stresses evoking such patient responses as irritability, withdrawal, sadness, and excessive preoccupation with the body (Rachman and Philips, 1980). For a successful adaptation, patients must be extensively prepared for the transfer from a relatively safe, secure environment to an anxiety-provoking and potentially painful one. Research suggests that preparation of the patient for a stressful event can reduce anxiety and facilitate recovery from illness and surgery (Janis, 1971). The process of preparation should include clarification of the patient's feelings about the experience, prediction and understanding of his sense of vulnerability, and support for his efforts to reduce his physical and psychological distress. The stress and anxiety that stem from the patient's unfamiliarity with the hospital environment and lack of adequate information concerning his medical problem can be relieved in part by reassurance. Providing information about the purpose and rationale of scheduled medical procedures and the results and implications of the findings will do much to alleviate anxiety. Nursing and medical staff occupy the central position in giving patients this information. The benefits of personal communication for the patient are far greater than those of printed material: Patients enjoy and need the opportunity to express their concerns and ask questions at the moment they arise.

Attention to the psychological needs of the patient is essential throughout treatment, before, during, and after hospitalization. Anxiety often results from lack of knowledge about the hospital routine, staff responsibilities, and personal identity and function within the hospital setting. Patients who are not severely ill routinely experience very marked anxiety when they are surrounded by those who are. Psychological distress, pain, and loss of self-esteem are common responses to hospitalization that are not necessarily associated with medical illness. Hospital staff can meet the patient's psychological needs in five ways: (1) by encouraging emotional expression; (2) by reinforcing behaviors that acknowledge the reality of the illness; (3) by providing relevant information about the illness and diagnostic procedures; (4) by building a warm, supportive relationship among patients and all staff; and (5) by preparing the patients for the future.

Patients are frequently anxious about recovery, disability, and family issues. Patients may be attention-seeking, demanding, depressed, or a combination of these, but the two most common coping mechanisms among hospitalized medical patients are withdrawal and excessive talking. Physiological manifestations of anxiety (e.g., sweating, palpitations, hyperventilation) may also occur periodically. Although antianxiety and antidepressant medication may occasionally be effective, helping the patient verbalize his concerns and examine his feelings may be a more appropriate method of decreasing tension and enabling the patient to perceive his problems realistically. Medication reinforces passivity on the part of the patient; talking about his concerns encourages a more active, problem-solving approach, which implies that the patient is capable of managing his life even during illness. Thus, a healthy self-image is bolstered, one that will foster a more successful adaptation after the illness. Allowing the patient to verbalize his worries within a supportive, accepting relationship, together with giving him information about procedures and hospital routines, will reduce anxiety, strengthen coping mechanisms, and help to establish a reasonable adjustment to the illness and hospital routine.

Hospitalized patients who lose a body part through surgery experience a sense of loss – as if a part of them had actually died. Body image is abruptly altered, and a grief reaction occurs that is likely to last for a significant period. Mastectomy patients, for example, feel mutilated and unfeminine. Anxieties about their husbands' love for them and acceptability to others are paramount. Depression and social isolation are two common, acute responses to mastectomy. In evaluating the severity of the grief reaction, health care professionals must consider the patient's psychological strengths and weaknesses while realistically assessing the illness and loss. Staff can best cope with the patient by communicating full acceptance of her thoughts and feelings, listening in an empathic way, and allowing her to work through her concerns, simultaneously permitting "time-outs" in which she is encouraged to avoid illness-related topics. Engel (1971) described three stages of the grief reaction: (1) disbelief – the refusal to accept the loss; (2) awareness – acknowledgment of the loss, often accompanied by apathy, fatigue, and anger; and (3) resolution – completion of the grief reaction accompanied by acceptance and adaptation. Patients who know they will lose a body part can best face the event by reviewing it before it occurs and airing their feelings and concerns. Talking is one way patients are able to reduce anxiety and mobilize psychological strength to cope with the stress of their loss.

COMMUNICATION BETWEEN
CLINICIAN AND PATIENT

The hospital staff has significant opportunities to deal with the patient's feelings regarding his illness, but the clinician responsible for the patient, usually the physician, occupies a primary role. A collaborative relationship between physician and patient should be established from the first contact. It should enable the patient to take as much responsibility for his own behavior as possible as well as maximize the probability of compliance with the prescribed treatment plan. As part of the collaborative relationship, the clinician must acknowledge that his feelings about the patient will be expressed, whether subtly or more obviously. Maintaining a positive tone in the initial assessment and examination facilitates the information-gathering process, increases the patient's motivation to cooperate with the clinician's recommendations for prophylactic or therapeutic regimens, and communicates respect and empathy for the patient. Enelow and Swisher (1972) stated that an empathic response consists of reflecting the patient's feelings as they are implied in his words, accepting the patient as an individual in his own right, and according him respect and dignity. The clinician must pay attention to the patient's feelings about his illness or other difficulty, regardless of whether the patient actually raises psychological issues for discussion. Building a positive working relationship is a crucial goal from the first contact.

Annon (1974a) described four levels of treatment for psychophysiological disorders or medical problems with significant psychological overlay that are geared to the needs and concerns of the patient: (1) the patient is given "permission" to have the problem of which he complains; (2) he provides for the clinician specific factual information relevant to the problem; (3) the clinician offers concrete suggestions to help the patient overcome the presenting problem; and (4) for problems that remain unresolved, additional forms of intervention, including behavioral strategies like social skills training, cognitive training, assertiveness training, desensitization, and relaxation, are used. Physicians faced with a highly anxious patient may find knowledge of relaxation and desensitization procedures useful even though the anxiety is frequently complex. Necessary aspects of the treatment process include changing the reinforcement patterns or contingencies in the patient's natural environment, teaching coping skills, and helping the patient's family to deal with the difficulty. Family members may need to modify their actions so as to help maintain the behavior the patient has just learned.

PSYCHIATRIC CONSULTATION

At times, the health care professional with primary responsibility for the patient must consider referring the patient for consultation with a psychiatrist. Epidemiological studies (Lipowski, 1975; Lipowski, 1967; and Moffic and Paykel, 1975) have found that 30–60 percent of a medical in-patient sample had a concomitant psychiatric disorder; only 2–12 percent of those patients were actually referred to a psychiatrist. The low percentage can be attributed in part to the feeling of many clinicians that psychiatrists offer little help to patients; their suggestions are perceived as vague and difficult to put into practice. Another common criticism is that psychiatric consultations upset patients because they imply that patients must be "crazy." The referring clinician may also be worried about potential critical review of his initial activity with the patient. These concerns are apt to arise when especially difficult patients are referred for psychiatric consultation.

Certain goals, however, can be achieved through consultation. Referral questions should be well thought-out and worded concisely. One goal of consultation is to encourage patient compliance. Van Dyke, Rice, Pallett, and Leigh (1980) investigated the relationship between the psychiatric consultant and the staff. Most studies assessing the effects of consultation on compliance have focused on patient satisfaction. The outcome is considered successful if compliance increases when the patient perceives the connection between the presenting difficulty and his lifestyle. These studies evaluated only those psychiatric consultations where physicians made formal requests for such consultation. Fifty-one percent of the study patients were depressed. By comparison, 20–30 percent of medical patients and 65 percent of cardiac intensive care patients are depressed (Lipowski, 1975; Lipowski and Kurlakos, 1972). For the patients in the study by Van Dyke et al., several treatments were used, including antidepressant medication and supportive psychotherapy. An overall compliance rate of 90 percent was found; this appears to be a somewhat biased finding, as the sample consisted only of those formally referred for consultation. The investigators concluded that medical staff members generally delay their requests for psychiatric evaluation so that when they do ask for help they are desperate and are more likely to comply. The results of the study also indicate that a high level of satisfaction with treatment outcome was noted mutually between patients and staff. Psychiatric consultation appeared to have a positive effect on the clinical care of these medical patients.

A second benefit of psychiatric consultation is that it can facilitate recognition by health care workers involved with the patient of present and potential areas of emotional conflict. Patients routinely respond emotionally to illness and hospitalization; acute anxiety, depression, confusion, and extreme dependency are not unusual. The staff, on the other hand, is more concerned with the target physical symptoms and the necessary treatment. These concerns may lead to conflict, problems in communication, and personality clashes between patients and staff. Consultation with a psychiatrist can help staff members cope with the patient and alter their response to the patient and the treatment management plan, if necessary. This approach is helpful for behaviors that appear to be based on emotional reactions to illness and maintained by the patterns of response by significant others. Data from work by Van Dyke, Rice, Pallett, and Leigh (1980) reveal that medical staff members can in fact alter their stance if this change produces improved relationships with the patient and less disruptive behavior. Thus, the staff can provide important reinforcement of the modification of maladaptive patient behavior.

It is important, then, that psychiatric consultation be available for patients demonstrating frank psychiatric symptomatology for whom medication and acute care (e.g., psychiatric hospitalization) may be indicated. Elderly medical patients, for example, may experience an acute sense of confusion, disorientation, and depression as they must face the reality of their impairment resulting from illness or surgery. Medication is sometimes appropriate for such patients, particularly when the symptoms interfere with their ability to tolerate the medical care they need. Difficult behavior on the part of patients that makes them a management problem for staff also constitutes appropriate reasons for such consultation although, in this case, the consultation is directed to staff to bring about changes in patient behavior. Medication is helpful for patients whose symptoms are severe and not amenable to behavioral intervention. Many patients with psychophysiological illness or chronic pain are depressed and require a thorough evaluation of their need for medication. Medication is often requested for a "difficult" patient, that is, one the staff finds hard to manage, but premature or inappropriate use of medication should be discouraged; it is apt to blur the symptom picture and confound the diagnostic formulation.

THE ROLE OF THE PSYCHOLOGIST

Psychologists are increasingly involved in nonpsychiatric medical settings. Personality assessment continues to be a major responsibility, but studying and treating the impact of emotions on physical health and the psychological consequences of medical illness are also in the domain of the psychologist. Such factors as socioeconomic status, stress, and attitude toward illness may both increase susceptibility to and aggravate various physical ailments. In both cases, it is the psychologist's job to determine the psychosocial factors that relate to either the development or the exacerbation of various types of physical illness and to maximize treatment efficiency by ensuring that premorbid personalty traits are taken into consideration. The overall goal is to understand the relevance of personality factors to the current medical illness.

Occasionally medical patients are transferred to the psychiatric service. Such transfer may be necessitated by acute psychopathological episodes or the detection of psychological difficulties that for some reason were not apparent during the original admission work-up or in the course of hospitalization. Most psychological consultations tend to occur with two types of patients: those having psychological difficulty related to either the stress of illness and hospitalization or real problems arising during the course of hospitalization, and those requiring assessment and treatment of psychophysiological or stress-tension disorders (several of these were discussed in Chapter 3). Psychologists are well qualified to deal with both groups.

One specific group of patients, those with chronic pain syndrome, are frequently referred for psychiatric evaluation because of obvious dependency and uncertainty about the etiology of the disorder. Pain patients may show no overt signs of psychiatric disturbance during the initial interview and mental status examination. Psychiatrists are reluctant to prescribe psychotropic medication prematurely if depression or functional disorder is not present. Many

chronic pain patients experience a reactive depression as a consequence of feeling helpless and unable to elicit positive regard from
their environment. McLean (1976) noted that to be effective, treatment programs for depressed patients must have the capacity for
teaching skills in which depressives are deficient – interpersonal communication, behavioral productivity, social interaction, assertiveness,
decision making, problem solving, and cognitive self-control. Psychologists are trained to evaluate the suitability of patients for such a
program and to institute therapy.

Another modality that psychologists use is family counseling.
Early intervening in the family is one way to keep a maladaptive
behavior pattern from becoming chronic. One popular theoretical
framework underlying family intervention is the systems approach
(Bowen, 1961), which views the symptoms of one member as part of
a number of events involving all family members and their interactions. The etiology and manner of presentation of problems are
viewed as family-based rather than belonging to any one individual.
No one person is labeled the "identified patient." Rather, one
person's behavior is viewed as an aspect of the family's behavior.
Consider a woman who has just had open-heart surgery and her husband who nags her to avoid activity and stress. She becomes depressed because of her sense of incapacitation and isolation from her
usual routine, but, knowing that her husband acts only to protect her
from potential illness, she fears that he will be hurt if she reveals her
negative feelings to him. A circular process is set up in which the husband nags and the patient becomes depressed. Trying to be more active in a compensatory way only causes her husband to nag her more
vociferously to curtail her activity. The husband-wife dysfunction
gradually escalates. Family counseling for this couple would mean
identifying the connections between their feelings and behaviors and
modifying the communications between them to make them more
clear and direct.

There are two major steps in the family counseling process. The
first is interviewing the entire family, with all members present, including the elderly and infants. Information about the members' jobs,
backgrounds, and daily activities is collected. The psychologist notes
which members are the responders and which ones are the
withdrawers, the pattern of verbal and nonverbal interaction, and the
seating arrangement the family selects. It is particularly important to
solicit each member's independent perception of the presenting

problem, noting who first raises the issue and who is labeled the patient by the family.

The second step is to identify the disturbed interactional patterns. Dysfunctional patterns include singling out one member as the cause of all the family problems, labeling a member or members as inappropriate or inaccurate, and bringing in a third-person scapegoat to enable two other members to resolve a difficulty. Important goals of counseling are: (1) the redefinition of the problem as family-based; (2) alteration of the labeling process and the labels themselves; and (3) avoidance of scapegoating so that no family member blames any other member or talks for any other member. Firm limit-setting by the therapist to encourage family members to talk to each other rather than through the therapist reduces the family tendency to criticize and find fault and enhances the possibility of change. It is essential that labels such as "a good child," "perfectly normal," and "typical man (woman)" be eradicated, because they curtail family change and growth. The labeling process may be supported by an entire family, but an individual member sometimes must take responsibility for its maintenance. Consider the child who is labeled "bad." It is likely that reinforcement of bad behaviors is occuring; for example, he may seem to keep his parents together because they interact only around his bad behaviors. The child must gradually learn to see that he doesn't have to keep his parents together by staying "bad." If his parents argue, the child may have an episode of hyperventilation. Their tendency may be to stop arguing and attend to the child. Thus, by bringing the child into their interaction, they never confront or resolve their anger. It is important to encourage the parents to remain a dyad, perhaps by delaying discussion of their disparate feelings until the child is asleep. Some physicians may feel comfortable meeting with the family for a few evaluative sessions, but prolonged contact necessitates referral to a psychologist or psychiatric social worker.

Psychological consultations in the hospital setting are preferably instituted formally with the cooperation of the full staff, but they may also be done occasionally via brief phone exchanges or notes in the patient's chart. Psychologists approach consultations with medical patients within either a behavioral or a psychodynamic framework. An example of each follows.

An Example of Behavioral Assessment in Medicine. Two patients were hospitalized for treatment of acute leukemia. Both were in isolation because of a loss of resistance to disease and infection as a result of chemotherapy. Both showed symptoms for which physical examination and laboratory tests were unable to find any organic or physical cause. Patient A developed a deep, raspy cough; patient B's symptom was excessive regurgitation of saliva, or retching.

A behavioral analysis was conducted by the psychologist in both cases. The first step involved naturalistic observation. Audiotape recordings of the symptoms were obtained and provided a baseline of the frequency of occurrence of the symptoms. Then, to determine whether the presence of staff members evoked the symptomatic behaviors, nurses entered the rooms of the patients and interacted naturally with the patients. Under the baseline conditions for patient A, the symptom occurred 25 percent of the time when the patient was alone and 75 percent of the time when a nurse was present. The proportions were similar for patient B. These results were statistically significant. It was concluded that in both cases the symptoms were under the stimulus control of the ward nurses.

Intervention involved extinction (ignoring of symptoms) and differential reinforcement (social attention) by the nurses. For example, nurses were instructed to follow their usual procedures but not to mention the target symptom or to stay in the room if the symptom occurred (once the required nursing treatment was completed). This was straightforward extinction procedure: If the nurses' responses to the patient were somehow reinforcing the symptom, then ignoring them should eliminate the reinforcement and, eventually, the symptoms. Next, a differential reinforcement procedure was used: Nurses were told to remain in the patients' rooms and to talk with the patients for ten minutes whenever the target symptoms ceased or did not occur. Thus, reinforcement contingencies were altered; now, *nonoccurrence* of the symptoms was being reinforced through increased attention from the nurses.

Immediately following this intervention, the observed probabilities of occurrence of the behavioral symptoms were reassessed. This time, patient A emitted the symptom 12 percent of the time that he was alone and 14 percent of the time that a nurse was present, a significant change from pre-intervention probabilities. Results were similar for patient B. Follow-up studies at two weeks and six months revealed neither recurrence of the symptoms nor development of new symptoms.

Before the behavior modification program was initiated, the symptoms of both patients were under the inadvertent stimulus control of the ward nurses. Following the behavioral assessment, an intervention was planned that eliminated the symptoms within two weeks. While the symptoms of both patients were initially side effects of the chemotherapy, they had become operant behaviors emitted primarily under the control of certain social reinforcement contingencies. This study provides a good example of the way in which the intensive care environment can produce real behavioral problems. It also provides an example of how a careful behavioral assessment can suggest a successful intervention (Redd, 1980: 448– 455).

An Example of Psychodynamic Thinking in Medicine. Psychological consultation was requested for a man who had suffered a myocardial infarction, his second in the last four years, and who had recently transferred from the cardiac intensive care unit to a medical floor. He was a 45-year-old self-employed businessman, described by the nurse as a classical Type A personality – hostile, competitive, unable to relax, loud and pressured in speech, impatient with staff, and unable to reduce his business involvements during his convalescence. He was bossy and often uncooperative with the staff. He failed to follow dietary and activity restrictions in the hospital, as he had before this most recent coronary event. The nursing staff felt frustrated in their efforts to help him and considered his behavior reckless and self-destructive. A social worker who had interviewed him reported that he was extremely fatalistic about his condition and unwilling to change his lifestyle, even though it would increase (admittedly by an unknown amount) his chances of a longer life. He had told her that he had changed radically following the onset of coronary heart disease (CHD) – on several occasions, for example, he had become so angry that he struck his children or his wife and then cried all night.

There is much interest at present in using behavior modification techniques to alter various aspects of Type A behavior. (There is little evidence, however, that such interventions produce long-term change, and no evidence yet that altering Type A behavior will reduce incidence or recurrence of CHD). Among the types of intervention that have been suggested are relaxation procedures, response-cost techniques that penalize the respondent for specific Type A activities, schedule engineering to minimize situations that might elicit Type A behavior, and thought stopping to aid relaxation. All of these depend on a cooperative subject. A Skinnerian, always sensitive to the influence of the environment on behavior, would doubtless observe that men in our society are positively reinforced for Type A behavior by material success and the admiration of their peers. To reduce such behavior, one must modify the existing reinforcement contingencies, a difficult task at both individual and societal levels.

The psychodynamic approach proceeds toward intervention from a different set of assumptions. It might postulate in this case that the patient's lifelong Type A behavior results in part from anxiety, that it is motivated by a need to escape anxiety by asserting control over all aspects of the environment and by compensating for underlying feelings of inadequacy by constant striving for outward signs of worth and achievement. As long as the patient remained healthy, this adaptation was successful from the standpoints of the individual and society, if not from a mental health standpoint. But once the man fell ill, he was suddenly helpless. He was in a situation whose outcome he could not control and depended on others for his survival, whereas previously others had been dependent on him. He admitted to the social worker that he had felt inadequate as a man since his illness began, suggesting a partial regression to a childlike form of thinking that equates the part (the disease, in this case) with the whole (the whole man).

This phenomenological account helps us begin to see how this man experiences his current illness and gives us some hunches as to why he behaves as he does. Much of his behavior may be seen as an attempt to proceed as if nothing had happened—"business as usual." He did not deny that he was ill, but he did seem to be denying the severity of his illness and the possible adverse affects of his behavior on his health. In other words, psychologically it was more important for this man to carry on as before than to be a cooperative patient. Being a cooperative patient would mean evoking all the anxiety, feeling of inadequacy, and now, too, the fear of dying for which he had spent a career trying to compensate. The incidents with his family show that he has aggressive impulses as well. Illness temporarily prevented the channeling of hostile impulses through Type A behavior, his previous mode of adjustment. Angry and inadequate, but without his customary defenses, he was unable to modulate his feelings and struck out with little provocation.

Given this background, a psychodynamically oriented practitioner may become uncomfortable with his behavioral colleagues' readiness to intervene to alter behavior. Behavior, for the psycho-dynamically oriented, represents a compromise between impulse and defense. It is a solution, however maladaptive, to a problem and one that is not changed easily. It was clear that in this case the patient would resist direct efforts to get him to change.

Recommendations by the psychologist to the nurses were as follows: If the patient engaged in obviously life-threatening behavior he would have to be stopped by direct order from the physician, by confrontation, or by any means possible. But if, as all agreed at this point, he was merely acting foolishly, then one might attempt more indirect methods of change, all the while remembering that any change would be modest. It would be important not to challenge him and to serve as a consultant with regard to his health, leaving the ultimate responsibility for change with him. He seemed to talk readily and honestly to the social worker (who had psychiatric social work training) and it seemed best for her to continue to meet with him to ventilate his concerns, in the hope that, as he heard himself talk, he would put into words some of the feelings he was experiencing and would not need to engage in such self-destructive acts. In other words, this man, who was neither psychotic nor suicidal, might be able to attenuate some of his more pathological conduct if only permitted to get in touch with his feelings. Time and distance from his recent myocardial infarction were viewed as perhaps further attenuating his more flagrant Type A behavior. Finally, support of the staff's effort, acknowledgment that such patients are indeed frustrating to work with, and encouragement of more modest treatment goals were offered (Zeldow, 1980). Thus, although behavior modification techniques are often helpful, psychodynamic intervention can frequently facilitate catharsis and aid in the improvement in the patient's physical status. Such an approach, in fact, is often useful for bright, reflective people who relish interpersonal contact as a means of support and change.

THE BEHAVIORAL MEDICINE UNIT

Patients with psychophysiological and stress-tension disorders, along with such associated problems as anxiety and pain, are commonly hospitalized for treatment on psychiatric floors. There are three major criticisms of this current practice: (1) physicians often hesitate to refer patients with known organic illness, undiagnosed somatic complaints, or vague psychological symptoms for evaluation in a psychiatric setting because of patient anxiety about and resistance to interaction with psychiatric patients; (2) patients with these disorders infer incorrectly that a psychological treatment approach means that their problems are "only psychological" and tend as a result to be uncooperative in treatment; and (3) psychiatric units cannot be sufficiently flexible as to incorporate the extensive assessment and treatment programs required for these patients when they are also responsible for managing acute and chronic psychiatric disturbance. The need for a less conventional setting for the diagnosis and treatment of these kinds of medical and stress-related disorders is clear.

One such unit has been organized at the Dartmouth-Hitchcock Medical Center in Hanover, New Hampshire, to aid physicians in working with these groups of patients. Patients who have medical illnesses with a significant psychological or psychophysiological component in which anxiety predominates are eligible for admission. The organic and psychological components of illness can thereby be considered in a medical setting in which assessment and treatment are based on learning and behavioral strategies.

The behavioral medicine unit combines the medical model of disease and the behavioral approach to psychological symptomatology. There are two phases of evaluation. The first is an initial assessment, lasting four or five days, of newly admitted patients. It includes: (1) psychological history, mental status and physical examination; (2) a behaviorally oriented interview; (3) psychophysiological assessment (the history or current status of the chief complaint); (4) nursing interviews and observations of behavior; (5) psychological testing; and (6) monitoring of baseline target behaviors by the patient. Interviewing family members provides information about their view of the patient's problem and their own patterns that reinforce his maladaptive behavior. Observation of the patient's capacity to cope with in vivo task situations—that is, situations that require problem solving or carrying out of a task—and a variety of interpersonal circumstances allows the staff to determine whether verbal self-reports of behavior repertoire match actual events. The patient's defense mechanisms and difficulties in specific aspects of interpersonal functioning become apparent to him as well as the staff, and the patient gradually becomes a sharp observer of his own behavior.

The second phase of the evaluation is the determination of psychophysiological variables. Measures are taken of the frontalis electromyogram (EMG) response, digital skin temperature, and heart rate to determine whether relaxation-biofeedback intervention is suitable, and if so, what would be the best site for intervention.

After the initial assessment, the appropriate treatment is instituted. Behavioral and medical intervention and traditional psychotherapy and counseling are all available and are employed when useful. The family is encouraged from the outset to be actively involved in the intervention program. The precise role of the family varies according to the patient's presenting complaint and his current needs as evaluated by the staff.

The medical atmosphere is emphasized by the hospital beds, white coats, traditional nursing uniforms, and daily physician rounds. The staff maintains a traditional medical stance with patients; interaction occurs primarily around illness-related issues—medication, for example. (This approach differs markedly from the notion of milieu, currently a popular treatment modality for psychiatric in-patients, in which the atmosphere of the outside world is maintained as far as possible and interaction around issues of coping rather than medication is encouraged.) The patient's belief that his physical symptoms result from organic illness, which can be treated in a medical environment, is reinforced by the characteristics of the unit. This reinforcement facilitates the therapeutic alliance. The milieu is de-emphasized as a therapeutic tool. The strategy of enhancing the medical aspects of the unit does several things for the patient. It acknowledges the validity of his complaint; it communicates to him that stress outside the hospital can exacerbate his symptoms; and it demonstrates to him the need for detailed assessment to provide the basis for designing a therapeutic stress management program. This rationale tends to be acceptable to patients because it corresponds to their common-sense understanding of illness. Once the patient acknowledges the role of stress in his disorder, he can accept the need for a comprehensive behavioral assessment. The medical symbols around him allow and strengthen the belief that he is medically ill. Yet, the explanation about stress given him by the staff clarifies in a supportive way the role of psychological factors in his symptoms and helps to minimize hostility and defensiveness.

It is notoriously difficult to find an appropriate in-patient treatment facility for this group of patients. Because they are not necessarily psychologically incapacitated, at least initially, they cannot always be admitted to psychiatric units. And, as noted above, psychiatric units do not offer truly appropriate treatment programs for these patients. Nevertheless, their life patterns may be tremendously disrupted by such symptoms as anxiety and pain. These patients have often reached an impasse with their physicians: Extensive work-up has either revealed no organic basis for the complaint or yielded a diagnosis for which no medical or surgical intervention can provide relief. These patients are usually frequent visitors to their physicians' offices and local emergency rooms. They undergo many diagnostic and treatment procedures without benefit; this frequently leads to "doctor-shopping" and frustration for both patients and physicians. One special benefit of the treatment in a behavioral unit is that patients learn to incorporate new coping skills into their behavioral repertoires and to give up inappropriate illness behavior.

SUMMARY

Many patients faced with the stress of a significant medical illness and hospitalization could benefit from psychological and behavioral intervention. Although the structured hospital setting may appear to offer many resources for such intervention, physicians' requests for consultation do not always address themselves to important issues such as anxiety, pain, loss of self-esteem, withdrawal, depression, and excessive talking, common responses to the stress of hospitalization. Occasionally, antianxiety and antidepressant medication may be helpful. Medication, however, reinforces the patient's sense of passivity and helplessness in dealing with his problems. Anxiety can more effectively be reduced by encouraging the patient to verbalize his concerns, by providing the appropriate factual information about his illness and diagnostic procedures, by building a supportive relationship between patient and staff, and by preparing the patient for the future. It is important that the patient start to develop coping mechanisms while he is hospitalized as a basis for adjustment once he is released.

It is essential that the patient have a collaborative relationship with his physicians and nurses. If the clinician is sensitive to the psychological needs of the patient and acknowledges their importance, the patient is more likely to feel understood and to comply with the prescribed treatment regimen. The behavioral aspects of a psychophysiological disorder, including the precise context in which it occurs, reinforcement contingencies, and issues of secondary gain, must receive attention. Physicians faced with a highly anxious patient may find relaxation training helpful as an initial temporary intervention. Because anxiety is invariably a complex reaction, a full behavioral assessment is needed to provide a basis for developing additional behavioral strategies.

Psychiatrists and psychologists are available to consult with hospital staff. Requests for psychiatric consultation should be made for patients with flagrant psychiatric symptoms that may require acute care (e.g., psychotropic medication, in-patient psychiatric care). In particular, depression in medical and surgical patients is often so severe that psychiatric intervention is necessary. Despite the stigma commonly attached to such treatments, referral is especially important when psychiatric symptoms interfere with the delivery of appropriate medical care and the current and posthospital adjustment. Both work with staff members to help them cope more effectively with a patient and direct professional contact with the patient himself are potential forms of consultation.

Psychologists are particularly well equipped to intervene in psychological and stress-tension disorders and in psychological problems resulting from the stress of medical illness. In the case of psychological and stress-tension disorders the goal of intervention is to demonstrate the connection of the somatic manifestations of the disorder to the behavior and patterns of reinforcement that maintain the problem. A careful behavioral assessment can suggest a successful intervention program to alter maladaptive behavior. A psychodynamic formulation is sometimes more appropriate in treating patients experiencing difficulty in coping with medical illness and hospitalization. The constraints imposed by illness and hospitalization are viewed in this framework as preventing the patient from engaging in his routine, comfortable mode of adjustment.

Patients with psychophysiological and stress-tension disorders are commonly hospitalized for treatment on psychiatric floors, although they are not appropriate psychiatric admissions. The need for units to diagnose and treat these patients has been acknowledged, but few have been built. One such unit currently in operation emphasizes the medical aspects of the disorder while behavioral assessment and intervention make up the primary approach to treatment. In particular, intervention focuses on the identification and alteration of psychological and behavioral contingencies that maintain or exacerbate the illness. The behavioral medicine unit is a comprehensive facility in which patients can accept the role of stress in the presenting problem and participate in a structured treatment designed to help them replace the maladaptive illness behavior with more appropriate coping skills.

BIBLIOGRAPHY

Annon, J. S. *The behavioral treatment of sexual problems. I. Brief therapy.* Honolulu: Enabling Systems, 1974a.

_____. *The behavioral treatment of sexual problems. II. Intensive therapy.* Honolulu: Enabling Systems, 1974b.

Bandura, A. Self-efficacy: Towards a unifying theory of behavioral change. *Psychological Review,* 1977, 84:191–215.

Bowen, M. Family psychotherapy. *American Journal of Orthopsychiatry,* 1961, 31:40–60.

Brockway, B. S. Behavioral medicine in family practice: A unifying approach for the assessment and treatment of psychosocial problems. *Journal of Family Practice,* 1978, 6:545–552.

Budzynski, T. H. Biofeedback procedures in the clinic. In L. Birk (Ed.), *Seminars in psychiatry,* 5 vols. (New York: Grune and Stratton, 1973), 5:415–428.

Davidson, R. J., and Schwartz, G. F. The psychobiology of relaxation: A multiprocess theory. In D. I. Mostofsky (Ed.), *Behavior control and modification of physiological activity* (Englewood Cliffs, New Jersey: Prentice-Hall, 1976), pp. 206–243.

Ellis, A. *Reason and emotion in psychotherapy.* New York: Lyle Stuart, 1962.

Enelow, A. J., and Swisher, S. N. *Interviewing and patient care.* New York: Oxford University Press, 1972.

Engel, G. Sudden rapid death during psychological stress, folklore or folk wisdom? *Annals of Internal Medicine,* 1971, 74:771.

Goldfried, M. R., and Merbaum, M. (Eds.). *Behavior change through self-control.* New York: Holt, Rinehart and Winston, 1973.

Janis, I. *Stress and frustration.* New York: Harcourt Brace Jovanovich, 1971.

Jenkins, C. D. Social and epidemiological studies in psychosomatic disease. *Psychiatric Annals,* 1972, 1:8–21.

Johnson, B. C., Karvnes, T. M., and Epstein, F. H. Longitudinal change in blood pressure in individuals, families and social groups. *Clinical Science Molecular Medicine,* 1973, 45:35–45.

Katz, R., and Zlutnick, R. *Behavior therapy and health care: Principles and applications.* New York: Pergamon Press, 1975.

Leigh, H., and Reiser, M. F. Major trends in psychosomatic medicine: The psychiatrist's evolving role in medicine. *Annals of Internal Medicine,* 1977, 87:223–239.

Lewinsohn, P. M. The behavioral study and treatment of depression. In M. Hersen, R. Eisler, and P. M. Miller (Eds.), *Progress in behavior modification* (New York: Academic Press, 1975), pp. 9–64.

Ley, P. Psychological studies of doctor-patient communication. In S. Rachman (Ed.), *Contributions to medical psychology,* vol. 1 (Oxford: Pergamon Press, 1977), 1–42.

Liberman, R. P., and Raskin, D. C. Depression: A behavioral formulation. *Archives of General Psychiatry,* 1971, 24:515.

Lipowski, Z. Review of consultation psychiatry and psychosomatic medicine. II. Clinical aspects. *Psychosomatic Medicine,* 1967, 24:201–224.

———. Psychiatry of somatic diseases: Epidemiology, patrogenesis, classification. *Comprehensive Psychiatry,* 1975, 16:105–124.

Lipowski, Z., and Kurlakos, R. Borderlands between neurology and psychiatry: Observations in a neurological hospital. *Psychiatric Medicine,* 1972, 3:137–147.

Lipowski, Z. J. Psychosomatic medicine in the 70's: An overview. *American Journal of Psychiatry,* 1977, 134:233–234.

McLean, R. Parental depression: Incompatible with effective parenting. In E. J. Mash, L. A. Hamerlynck, and L. C. Handy (Eds.), *Behavior modification in families* (New York: Brunner/Mazel, 1976), pp. 106–122.

Moffic, H., and Paykel, E. Depression in medical in-patients. *British Journal of Psychiatry,* 1975, 126:346–353.

Rachman, S. J., and Philips, C. *Psychology and behavioral medicine.* New York: Cambridge University Press, 1980.

Redd, W. R. Stimulus control and extinction of psychosomatic symptoms in cancer patients in protective isolation. *Journal of Consulting and Clinical Psychology,* 1980, 48:448–455.

Stone, R. A., and DeLeo, J. Psychotherapeutic control of hypertension. *New England Journal of Medicine,* 1976, 294:80–84.

Van Dyke, C., Rice, D., Pallett, P., and Leigh, H. Psychiatric consultation: Compliance and level of satisfaction with recommendations. *Psychotherapeutic Psychosomatics,* 1980, 33:14–24.

Weisman, A. D., and Worden, J. W. Psychosocial analysis of cancer deaths. *Omega: Journal of Death and Dying,* 1975, 6:61–75.

Zeldow, P. Fundamentals of behavior: Syllabus for lecture on personality theory. Unpublished manuscript, Rush Medical College, Chicago, 1980.

6

PRESENT STATUS AND
FUTURE DIRECTIONS

INTRODUCTION

There is a tendency to "oversell" behavioral medicine as a new field that can provide immediate cures for a variety of disorders that were previously resistant to treatment. Of greater significance than its ability to specify intervention techniques, however, is the incorporation into the field of behavioral medicine of the rigorous scientific method to focus on the behavioral aspects of medical problems and therapy (Agras, 1975). The knowledge that learning can play a significant role in causing and maintaining certain forms of illness and disease underlies the current emphasis on relating measurable activity to antecedent and environmental cues for behavior.

Two concepts, reinforcement and stimulus control, are basic to this formulation. Reinforcement consists of those events that determine the pattern of behavior. It can be direct: In the case of obesity, for example, if eating reduces tension, tension reduction would be a reinforcer of the eating behavior. Reinforcers are defined by their effects on the subsequent frequency of the immediately preceding behavior. The rate of emission of a behavior already in a person's repertoire can be readily increased by a reinforcing stimulus that follows it. This process is termed operant conditioning, and the reinforcing stimulus, an operant reinforcer. Biofeedback is a good example of a situation in which operant reinforcers (i.e., tones) are presented following a response close to the desired response (i.e., a gradual reduction in frontalis EMG). Stimulus control refers to the influence of the environment on behavior. A stimulus can affect behavior by its association with a particular reinforcer. A stimulus control analysis enables us to specify the manner in which the en-

111

vironment determines the problem behavior: It focuses on the identification of target behaviors and environmental events that are
related temporally to those behaviors. Behavioral strategies are formulated to modify these stimuli and to put them under the control of
the individual rather than of the environment.

CURRENT STATUS

Major themes in the behavioral medicine literature are: (1) intervention to modify problematic or maladaptive behavior; (2) the
behavior of the health care professional; (3) the use of behavioral
strategies to facilitate compliance with a prescribed medical regimen;
and (4) the prevention of illness.

Intervention

Extensive experimental work has demonstrated that behavioral
strategies are effective in the treatment of certain psychophysiological
and stress-tension disorders. These strategies are formulated for each
person following a complete behavioral assessment of relevant factors—personality style, premorbid psychopathology, interpersonal
support system, preoccupation with bodily functioning, psychosomatic correlates of disease, and probable responsiveness to intervention. Successful intervention flows from a good behavioral
assessment. In contrast to other therapeutic frameworks, such as the
psychodynamic model, assessment often constitutes a significant part
of intervention. For example, for an obese person, recording the
amount of food eaten and the circumstances in which the eating occurs for a two-week period provides baseline data on the presenting
problem of obesity; at the same time it functions as a self-monitoring
device that gives immediate feedback about the relationship between the target behavior of eating and the reinforcers of this behavior.

The primary goal of behavioral intervention is to alter present
maladaptive patterns of behavior. Several approaches have been described: self-monitoring, cueing, stimulus control, modification of incentives, and rehearsal. Many others exist, but they have not been
sufficiently subjected to scientific scrutiny. Biofeedback and relaxation are perhaps the most frequently researched behavioral
strategies. Following Miller's (1969) work, which demonstrated that

visceral responses could be shaped, interest arose in the behavioral etiology of psychophysiological disorders. Studies of the biofeedback process showed that behavioral models are relevant to physiological functions and emotional states. Biofeedback is the process by which behavior is gradually shaped to the desired criterion by arranging the consequences of each successive stage of the behavior. It has clearly been a worthwhile tool for the study of the psychophysiological disorders, but despite acclaim and support from clinicians and subjects alike, its merit as a reliable treatment technique has not been substantiated by well-controlled research investigations.

At least part of the enthusiasm for biofeedback appears to stem from its seeming objectivity: It focuses on a manifest symptom, so that it is unnecessary for the therapist to invade the subject's confidential, subjective thoughts, feelings, and concerns; it has a clearly defined goal—elimination of the symptom; it produces rapid improvement and "cure"; and it is useful for many kinds of people, personalities, and disorders. But although biofeedback is symptom-focused and provides highly objective criteria by which therapeutic progress can be assessed, it is not a cure-all that can be applied indiscriminately to everyone. People who have a precise localized somatic complaint with a prominent stress-tension component and who need mastery and self-control may be better suited for biofeedback than are those who are more passive and oriented toward immediate gratification.

More experimental investigation of biofeedback intervention is needed. Although research has shown promising results with some psychophysiological disorders—migraine, for example—well-designed studies of the outcome of treatment are required to substantiate the overwhelming number of subjective findings. Identification of the precise mechanisms by which biofeedback works is needed. Controlled clinical trials, including treatment groups, placebo control groups, and wait-list control groups (in which patients are told that they are on the waiting list for treatment, thereby ensuring that they receive no treatment), are recommended. In addition, the crucial issue of generalizability of successful results from the treatment setting to the subject's natural environment and the duration of treatment results must receive further attention. More baseline data on pretreatment functioning should be obtained and the follow-up should be extended to at least one year. Factors that enhance compliance behavior (i.e., the subject continuing to practice his newly learned response) during follow-up require clarification. And, finally, the applicability of biofeedback to both acute and chronic psychophysiological disorders needs to be understood given the long-term relative costs of long-term biofeedback and untreated illness.

Although biofeedback has become fairly well established as a clinical tool, it has been used for only about twenty years. Studies comparing biofeedback training and relaxation training demonstrate that neither has a consistent superiority over the other in treating psychophysiological disorder. Stress and other factors that lead to a certain physiological response need elucidation. A combined cognitive-biofeedback approach would focus on the modification of the subject's style of interaction with the environment before changing the specific physiological response that is indicative of the predisposing factor.

The efficacy of behavioral intervention and other approaches used to treat psychophysiological disorder has yet to be demonstrated. Further research must address itself to certain key issues.

1. Specification of events that precipitate psychophysiological disorder is needed; what is the rate of stress, alone or in combination with impaired physiological functioning, that produces the problem?
2. There are racial, sexual, and cultural differences in the incidence of headache (Adams, Feuerstein, and Fowler, 1980); do sociodemographic differences enter into the incidence of other psychophysiological disorders?
3. Pharmacological intervention is appropriate for treatment of migraine. Can medication be used prophylactically? In view of the documented side effects, systematic evaluation of drug therapy in both acute and chronic illness is necessary.
4. Carefully controlled studies of behavioral techniques, such as assertiveness training, desensitization, relaxation, and biofeedback, are needed to confirm their effectiveness.

Because studies have used varying definitions of psychophysiological disorder and different assessment approaches, it is difficult to evaluate and compare them. The definition of the disorder in question and the details about the method of assessment are most often constructed from subjective data offered by the patient and from the self-monitoring record (Adams, Feuerstein, and Fowler, 1980). It is essential that the latter include information about the frequency, intensity, and severity of the target behavior. Identification of the behavioral indices of the problem, including the degree of disability or handicap that results from the disorder, the amount of time taken off from work due to the disability, and the type and frequency of medication taken, is extremely useful for both the clinician and the patient.

Behavior of the Clinician

It is essential that the clinician maintain an empathic, attentive stance. Flexibility of approach is necessary. The physician, for example, who refers a migraine headache patient for biofeedback treatment can allay the patient's anxiety and build a sense of confidence in the procedure, at the same time acknowledging the patient's underlying sense of frustration and self-recrimination because of his perceived loss of self-control and his inability to work because of disabling pain. Thus, although as noted in Chapter 5, a psychodynamic formulation may at times provide a helpful framework for understanding the disorder, behavioral intervention may be the most rational treatment approach.

Compliance

The third theme is the use of behavioral techniques to maximize compliance with a prescribed treatment regimen, either medical or behavioral. Noncompliance is a serious problem (Counte and Christman, 1981) and one of particular importance when evaluating a behavioral intervention. During the follow-up period after the actual supervised intervention, the subject is asked to practice the intervention according to a schedule that has been arranged by the clinician and subject. The purpose of this practice is to generalize the successful treatment outcome among settings and over time. Insufficient practice or no practice at all is likely to expedite return of the presenting symptom. Conditions must be arranged, then, so as to maximize the potential for compliance with the prescribed practice routine.

Maintenance of therapeutic improvement, a difficult problem in all psychological-behavioral therapy, has been attempted in five different ways: (1) conditioning, (2) booster sessions, (3) reprogramming the environment, (4) self-control methods, and (5) symbolic operations. Conditioning is problematic because it does not consider the effects of significant intervening variables. Occasional appointments with the clinician during the follow-up phase for intervention, or booster sessions, are not consistently successful. Environmental supports are essential to the maintenance of therapeutic improvement. However, massive alteration of the environment to achieve the proper support and reinforcement is viewed as unmanageable and infeasible. Self-control methods appear worthwhile because they imply that the subject has taken the responsibility for his own behavior change, but they tend often to lead to lack of control once the reinforcements or external limits are withdrawn. And, finally, the use of one's imagination to rehearse coping behaviors in response to high-risk situations (symbolic operations) has proven helpful for bright individuals with adequate abstraction ability. Symbolic operations are less valuable for less intelligent and highly anxious people who are apt to experience some concretization of thought with stress. Thus, there are problems with all five approaches.

Attribution theory suggests that therapeutic improvement can be maintained if the patient attributes his improvement to his own competence and achievement rather than to an external agent. A problem exists, however: How can a weak treatment effect be created so that the patient can attribute his improvement to his own efforts? The patient's social skills and incentives for treatment and maintenance of successful outcome must be maximized. The patient's sense of efficacy should be cited as having major influence on his persistent efforts to engage in adaptive coping behaviors.

There are currently two popular ways to increase the probability of compliance behavior and behavior change. The first is to offer an intervention package comprising several behavioral strategies. This looks better because more than one type of treatment is involved. In this approach, the expectation of the subject that improvement will occur results in a self-fulfilling prophecy and thereby facilitates compliance behavior. The second technique consists of placing marked emphasis on self-control procedures. The assumption is that a patient who is involved exclusively with extensive, daily self-monitoring behavior will probably continue this behavior long after the active intervention period.

In either case, if treatment fails, it is important to clarify the circumstances in which the failure occurred, what behaviors were assumed following relapse, what constitutes recidivism, and how it can be measured. It is important for patients with a history of previous relapse to learn to recognize high-risk situations and respond appropriately to them before it is too late. Self-monitoring methods are recommended in such cases because they help the patient record the target behavior for a definite period and the context or situation in which it occurs (McFall, 1977). The patient can then easily see under what circumstances the behavior occurs most frequently. Following identification of high-risk situations, the patient can be taught to make discriminative responses to cues and change his behavior significantly.

Assessment by the clinician and the patient of the quality of coping mechanisms evoked in the face of a potentially threatening situation should also occur. An understanding of the patient's present and potential coping skills assists the clinician in planning treatment. Training in social skills is frequently combined with such fear-reduction techniques as desensitization and relaxation. Desensitization, which is based on the patient's level of current functioning, encourages him to practice his newly learned skills in a nonthreatening situation so that he can gradually integrate these skills into his lifestyle. Advice-giving is viewed as mechanical; the patient may adhere to the advice without understanding it. It is more effective to help the patient develop a general approach to his problem and engage in cognitive relabeling to promote a sense of self-efficacy. Problem-solving strategies (D'Zurilla and Goldfried, 1971; Goldfried and Davison, 1976) should be formulated to teach the appropriate skills needed to cope with problems that might arise. Lastly, building in specific times during the day for pleasurable activity—time-out—will show the patient the importance of self-reward and help build positive self-esteem. As the patient feels better about himself, he is more likely to comply with the treatment plan and to maintain his improvement.

Compliance has been presented as a complex set of behaviors requiring an equally sophisticated treatment approach. The clinician must take care to respond to the patient's questions in a direct, open way. The possibility that patients have ideas about treatment that conflict with the prescribed treatment regimen must be considered; such differences between the patient and clinician are best dealt with openly. Simplifying the treatment plan at the beginning and adding additional steps as the patient feels able to manage them is a helpful approach that avoids inflicting undue anxiety on the patient. Asking the patient to report or paraphrase instructions as they are given ensures that he truly understands them; hence, there is a greater chance of compliance. Clinicians should schedule mandatory follow-up sessions to track ongoing compliance behavior and detect early signs of noncompliance.

Prevention

The fourth and final theme is the prevention of illness. Prevention has not been considered in this volume, but a few words about its importance are in order. Prevention involves the modification of certain aspects of lifestyle that may be maladaptive, for example, alcohol use, cigarette smoking, and insufficient or excessive physical activity. The impetus for prevention programs comes from the urgent need to change patterns of behavior that increase sharply the risk of chronic disease in the population (Pomerleau and Brady, 1979) and from economic considerations: Comparative cost-benefit analyses of prevention versus treatment of chronic illness show that prevention is cheaper (Kristen, Arnold, and Wynder, 1977).

SUMMARY AND DISCUSSION

Behavioral intervention is useful in the treatment and management of psychophysiological and stress-tension disorders as well as medical illnesses with significant psychophysiological consequences. The latter area is relatively new and has inspired excitement and enthusiasm. In this respect, the field of behavioral medicine encompasses health care psychology, the application of personality theory and principles of psychopathology to treatment of psychological difficulty accompanying medical illness. The enthusiasm for this field stems from recent work suggesting that recovery from medical illness is contingent in large part upon psychological health. The view that psychological stress can precipitate various illnesses is widely espoused, but it has not been established experimentally for most illnesses. Nevertheless, it suggests that there is probably a valid association, without implied causation, between stress, psychological status, and illness. This area is a promising one for researchers, although its current status is speculative at best. Nevertheless, the clinical utility of giving attention to the psychological needs and difficulties of patients before, during, and after illness has been shown repeatedly. What is needed now is corroboration of this observation by the objective data of competent experimental investigators.

Behavioral medicine is in a state of flux at present. Despite the popular enthusiasm, some researchers urge caution in applying behavioral principles to serious medical problems. They argue that "if the goal of behavioral technology is to modify the aberrant response (e.g., hypertension), one may be able to do so only to the extent possible within the limitations set by the pathology" (Schneiderman, Weiss, and Engel, 1979:xxiii–xxiv).

Behavioral science can make a strong contribution to medicine in five areas: (1) etiology, (2) the behavioral concomitants of physiological illness, (3) the basis for illness behavior and noncompliance, (4) long- and short-term psychological and behavioral response to illness, and (5) prevention of certain disorders through change in lifestyle. We need to develop more effective behavioral interventions that can be better integrated into the hospital setting. At this time, most programs utilizing behavioral strategies focus on a specific problem or disorder in a broad-based treatment center for behavioral problems. Methods of training professionals to practice behavioral medicine, as well as the kind of facility appropriate for treatment of patients with psychophysiological and stress-tension disorders, should be considered and training methods and treatment facilities that currently exist should be modified. The appealing interdisciplinary character of behavioral medicine will undoubtedly ensure its survival as a viable clinical and experimental field.

BIBLIOGRAPHY

Adams, E., Feuerstein, M., and Fowler, J. L. Migraine headache: Review of parameters, etiology, and intervention. *Psychological Bulletin,* 1980, 87:217–237.

Agras, S. Foreword. In R. C. Katz and S. Zlutnick (Eds.), *Behavior therapy and health care* (Elmsford, New York: Pergamon Press, 1975), pp. 1–5.

Counte, M. A., and Christman, L. P. *Interpersonal behavior and health care.* Boulder, Colorado: Westview Press, 1981.

Davidson, P. O., and Davidson, S. M. *Behavioral medicine: Changing health lifestyles.* New York: Brunner/Mazel, 1980.

D'Zurilla, T. J., and Goldfried, M. R. Problem-solving and behavior modification. *Journal of Abnormal Psychology,* 1971, 78:107–126.

Feldman, M. P., and Broadhurst, A. (Eds.). *Theoretical and experimental bases of the behavior therapies.* New York: John Wiley, 1976.

Feuerstein, M., and Schwartz, G. C. Training in clinical psychophysiology. *American Psychologist,* 1979, 32:560–567.

Goldfried, M. R., and Davison, G. C. *Clinical behavior therapy.* New York: Holt, Rinehart and Winston, 1976.

Kristen, M., Arnold, C., and Wynder, E. Health economics and preventive care. *Science,* 1977, 195:457–462.

Lipowski, Z. and Kurlakos, R. Borderlands between neurology and psychiatry. Observations in a neurological hospital. *Psychiatric Medicine,* 1972, 3:137–147.

McFall, R. M. Patterns of self-monitoring. In R. B. Stuart (Ed.), *Behavioral self-management: Strategies, techniques, and outcomes* (New York: Brunner/Mazel, 1977), pp. 196–214.

McNamara, J. R. (Ed.). *Behavioral approaches to medicine: Applications and analysis.* New York: Plenum, 1979.

Miller, N. Postscript in D. Singh and C. T. Morgan, *Current status of physiological psychology: Readings* (Monterey, California: Brooks/Cole Publishing Company, 1972), pp. 245–250.

———. Behavioral medicine as a new frontier: Opportunities and dangers. In J. M. Weiss (Ed.), *Proceedings of the National Heart and Lung Institute and working conference on health behavior: Bayse, Virginia, May 12–15, 1975* (Department of Health, Education, and Welfare Publication No. [NIH] 76-868) (Washington, D.C.: Government Printing Office, 1975).

———. Learning of visceral and glandular responses. *Science,* 1969, 163:434.

Pomerleau, O. F., and Brady, J. P. (Eds.). *Behavioral medicine: Theory and practice.* Baltimore: Williams and Wilkins, 1979.

Rigatelli, M., Curu, P., and De Berandinis, M. Some experiences of consultation–liaison psychiatry in a university hospital. *Psychotherapeutic Psychosomatics,* 1980, 33:1–6.

Schneiderman, N., Weiss, T., and Engel, B. Foreword. In O. F. Pomerleau and J. P. Brady (Eds.), *Behavioral medicine: Theory and practice* (Baltimore: Williams and Wilkins, 1979), pp. xxiii–xxiv.

Schwartz, G. C., and Weiss, S. M. What is behavioral medicine? *Psychosomatic Medicine,* 1977, 39:377–381.

Winefield, H. R., and Peay, M. Y. *Behavioral science in medicine.* Baltimore: University Park Press, 1980.

INDEX